The Practical Applicability of Toxicokinetic Models in the Risk Assessment of Chemicals

Proceedings of the Symposium *The Practical Applicability of Toxicokinetic Models in the Risk Assessment of Chemicals* held in The Hague, The Netherlands, 17–18 February 2000.
Organized by **OPDENKAMP - REGISTRATION & NOTIFICATION**
Koninginnegracht 23, 2514 AB The Hague, The Netherlands

Edited by

J. Krüse

H.J.M. Verhaar

and

W.K. de Raat

OpdenKamp Registration & Notification,
The Hague, The Netherlands

KLUWER ACADEMIC PUBLISHERS

DORDRECHT / BOSTON / LONDON

A C.I.P. Catalogue record for this book is available from the Library of Congress.

ISBN 1-4020-0934-8

Published by Kluwer Academic Publishers,
P.O. Box 17, 3300 AA Dordrecht, The Netherlands.

Sold and distributed in North, Central and South America
by Kluwer Academic Publishers,
101 Philip Drive, Norwell, MA 02061, U.S.A.

In all other countries, sold and distributed
by Kluwer Academic Publishers,
P.O. Box 322, 3300 AH Dordrecht, The Netherlands.

Printed on acid-free paper

Printed in the Netherlands.

CONTENTS

LIST OF CONTRIBUTORS

Dr. Bas J. Blaauboer
Associate Professor of Toxicology, Research Institute of Toxicology, Utrecht University, P.O. Box 80176, 3508 TD Utrecht, The Netherlands. Tel: +31 (0)30 2535330, Fax: +31 (0)30 2535077, e-mail: b.blaauboer@ritox.vet.uu.nl.

Dr. P.C. de Bragt, R. Tox.
Senior Officer of Public Health, Ministry of Health, Welfare and Sports, Inspectorate for Health Protection, P.O. Box 20350, 2500 EJ The Hague, The Netherlands. Tel: +31 (0)70 3405060, Fax: +31 (0)70 3405435.

Dr. Anette L. Bunge
Professor, Chemical Engineering and Petroleum Refining, Colorado School of Mines, Golden, CO 80401, USA. Currently at: Colorado State University, Fort Collins CO 80523, USA. Tel: +1 509-376-8462, Fax: +1 303-273-3730.

Dr. Richard A. Corley
Staff Scientist/Technical Group Leader, Chemical Dosimetry Group, Molecular Biosciences Group, Pacific Northwest National Laboratory, 902 Battelle Blvd, P.O. Box 999, MSIN P7-59, Richland, WA 99352, USA. Tel: +1 509-376-8462, Fax: +1 509-376-9064, e-mail: ra-corley@pnl.gov.

Dr. A.M. Jarabek
Research Toxicologist, National Center for Environmental Assessment, US-EPA, USA. Tel: +1 919-541-4577, Fax: +1 919-558-1213, e-mail: jarabek.Annie@epamail.epa

Dr. Pierre O. Droz, PD, CIH
Scientist, Institute for Occupational Health Sciences (IST), Lausanne University, Rue du Bugnon 19, CH-1005 Lausanne, Switzerland. Tel: +41 21-314-74, Fax: +41 21-314-7420, e-mail: pierre-olivier.Droz@inst.hospvd.ch.

Prof. Dr. V.J. Feron
Professor Emeritus, Utrecht University, Utrecht, The Netherlands. Tel: +31 (0)30-6959408, Fax: +31 (0)30 6960264, e-mail: v.jferon@freeler.nl.

Dr. Anette Kopp-Schneider

Senior Statistician,Central Unit Biostatistics, German Cancer Research Center, P.O. Box 101949, D-69009 Heidelberg, Germany. Tel: +49 6221-422-391, Fax: +49 6221-422-397, e-mail: kopp@dkfz-heidelberg.de.

Dr Jacob Krüse

OpdenKamp Registration & Notification, Koninginnegracht 23, 2514 AB The Hague, The Netherlands. Tel: +31 (0)70-426-0000, Fax: +31 (0)70-426-0001, e-mail: Krüse.j@oag.np.

Dr. John W. Nichols

Scientist, U.S. Environmental Protection Agency, National Health and Environmental Effects Laboratory, Mid-Continent, Ecology Division, 6201 Congdon Boulevard, Duluth, Minnesota, 55804, USA. Tel: +1 218-529-5160, Fax: +1 218-529-5003, e-mail: nichols.john@epa-gov.

Dr. K. de Raat

Director, OpdenKamp Registration & Notification, Koninginnegracht 23, 2514 AB The Hague, The Netherlands. Tel: +31 (0)70-426-0000, Fax: +31 (0)70-426-0001, e-mail: raatde.k@oag.nl.

Dr. Charles A. Timchalk, DABT

Staff Scientist, Molecular Biosciences Group, Chemical Dosimetry Group, Pacific Northwest Division, Batelle, Battelle Boulevard, Richland, WA., 99352, USA. Tel: +1 509-376-8462, Fax: +1 509-376-9064.
e-mail: charles.timchalk@pnl.gov.

Dr. Henk J.M. Verhaar

OpdenKamp Registration & Notification, Koninginnegracht 23, 2514 AB The Hague, The Netherlands. Tel: +31 (0)70-426-0000, Fax: +31 (0)70-426-0001, e-mail: Verhaar.h@oag.nl.

PREFACE

W.K.DE RAAT

Director OpdenKamp Registration & Notification, The Hague, The Netherlands

This symposium is concerned with a recognized problem area in especially regulatory toxicology. Effects in humans of the exposure to chemical substances are predicted from the results of toxicological studies with experimental animals. This prediction usually employs as a starting point an experimental exposure level of a certain animal species which lies just below the lowest level still causing an adverse effect in this species. The extrapolation from this so-called No Observed Adverse Effect Level (NOAEL) to a threshold level for human exposure is often solely based on the application of rather arbitrary extrapolation factors which are meant to cover all known and unknown differences between the animal in the experimental situation and man in real life. To ensure the outcome of extrapolation to be on the safe side, a worst-case strategy is followed, which simply means that large factors are chosen. Interestingly, usually no guarantee of safety can actually be given.

For a more realistic and tailor-made extrapolation, science-based factors are needed, taking into account the differences in kinetic and dynamic behaviour of a compound in different animal systems. Such factors might be derived on a case-by-case basis from:

- physicochemical properties of the substance;
- biochemical properties of the substance;
- general knowledge on the physiology determining toxicokinetics and metabolism in man and experimental animals.

To integrate this information in an adequate way, and incorporate it in predictions of safe levels, mathematical models are indispensable.

The obvious need for a more science-based extrapolation has resulted in extensive research efforts and a number of most promising toxicokinetic models. However, this has hardly resulted in a significant improvement of day-to-day risk assessment. A reason for this gap between developers of models and the risk assessors for whom they are ultimately intended might be a lack of communication. Clarity is needed on the tools wanted by the risk assessor, and information is needed on what is really possible with the models.

The organizing of this symposium was prompted by the concern about the arbitrary character of the extrapolation methods generally used and the unused possibilities of current toxicokinetic models. Experts in toxicokinetic modelling will demonstrate the possibilities and limitations of their models. It is hoped that this will trigger a discussion about the use of the models in day-to-day risk assessment.

1 THE PRACTICAL APPLICABILITY OF TOXICOKINETIC MODELS IN THE RISK ASSESSMENT OF CHEMICALS

V.J.FERON

Professor Emeritus, Utrecht University, Utrecht, The Netherlands

1.1 Introduction

In the early days of modern toxicology, say about half a century ago, major goals of toxicity studies were the detection of the critical adverse effect of the chemical and the establishment of the dose-effect/response curve including the "No-Observed-Adverse-Effect-Level" (NOAEL). Starting from the overall NOAEL, using body weight for scaling up between experimental animals and humans, and applying uncertainty factors to compensate for intra- and interspecies differences, a "safe" dose for humans was calculated. It is sad to observe that today too often we are still doing the same thing when recommending health-based exposure limits as the basis for setting standards.

Early on toxicologists realized that knowledge about both the movement and fate of a chemical within the body (toxicokinetics) and also about the mechanism underlying the toxicity, would be of great help for the interpretation of animal toxicity data with respect to human health risk assessment. The most solid comparison is when toxicokinetic data are available in experimental animals and man, allowing direct analysis of the potential health risk in humans. In the absence of human toxicokinetic data, physiological or compartmental models may be used for extrapolation of animal data to man (Feron *et al.*, 1990).

1.2 Underlying Principles of Toxicokinetic Models

Before discussing *"The Practical Applicability of Toxicokinetic Models in the Risk Assessment of Chemicals "*, we need to understand the underlying principles of the models in both biological and mathematical terms. The physiological approach relies on the scale-up between animals and man of such parameters as tissue volume and blood flow and on their relation to body weight. Assuming that the uptake from blood to tissue (extraction ratio) is a function of the chemical and thus independent of species, it is possi-

J. Krüse, H.J.M. Verhaar, and W.K. de Raat (eds.), The Practical Applicability of Toxicokinetic Models in the Risk Assessment of Chemicals, 1-6.

ble to derive (complex) models involving major organs. Alternatively and more pragmatically, the plasma toxicokinetics in various animal species may be fitted by compartmental modelling followed by scaling up empirically according to the body mass of the species examined and than to man (Renwick, 1989).

Application of such models would mean that risk assessment is based on scientific principles and understanding, implying that knowledge has been substituted for ignorance; ignorance which is often so terribly visible by the use of large uncertainty factors.

1.3 Lack of Data

Clearly, availability or lack of relevant data is one of the major factors related to the question whether or not toxicokinetic models are or can be applied in everyday risk assessment. Hazard identification including dose-effect/response curves and extrapolation of experimental data obtained in animals or humans to projected human exposure scenarios, constitutes the basis for the recommendation of so-called health-based intake levels or exposure limits. This first step in risk assessment or standard setting deals, and indeed should deal with toxicological data and health considerations only (Feron *et al.*, 1994; Feron, 1998). However, it is not exceptional that the toxicological data base, even for a widely used, high-production volume chemical, is too poor to justify the recommendation of an exposure limit. With too poor a data base, I do not mean lack of (sophisticated) toxicokinetic information but just insufficient straightforward toxicity data from repeat exposure studies such as for example a 4- or 13-week study in rats. Occasionally, some basic information about absorption, distribution , metabolism and/or elimination is available, but hardly ever to an extent and of a quality that would allow the data to be fed into a model for quantitative risk assessment. It is just the lack of information that precludes the use of any toxicokinetic model.

1.4 Use of Structure-Activity Relationships (SARs)

Toxicity is dependent on the chemical structure of a substance, its toxicokinetcs and its metabolic reaction pathways. Available metabolic pathways are usually dose dependent and, to a large extent, govern the magnitude of the toxic effect. Therefore, chemical structure, toxicokinetics, metabolic fate and dose are key elements of toxicity and play a crucial role in the safety evaluation of chemicals. Refinements of initial concepts of SARs were the result of increasing knowledge, and increased the confidence in predicting SARs. However, to my knowledge and in my experience, the use of SARs in safety evaluation of chemicals is rather limited. Has the use of SARs been sufficiently tried? Does it not work? Is it too complicated? Are SAR experts not interested or not involved in risk assessment? One thing I know for sure is that, except for the safety evaluation of flavouring substances, the risk assessments I have been involved in hardly ever used (quantitative) SARs. Indeed SARs play an important role in the safety evaluation of flavouring ingredients, and the use of SARs has been widely accepted for this category of food chemicals. This may be due mainly to large margins of safety as a consequence of the generally low intakes and often low toxicity of flavouring substances, and also to the production of "safe" metabolites (Munro *et al.*, 1999).

1.5 Standard Tests versus Compound-Specific studies

Guidelines and detailed protocols for standard tests are common in applied toxicology. For registration purposes defined sets of tests are required. These guidelines enabled worldwide standardization and harmonization of toxicity testing which was a good thing. However, the reverse side of the medal was discouragement of the development of alternative ways to develop toxicity profiles of chemicals. Thus, although the guidelines have been of great help, and still are key elements of toxicity testing, in my view we gradually have to get rid of rigid guidelines and predetermined sets of standard tests. The conduct of whole packets of such tests should be replaced by step-by-step investigations guided by decision trees for different production and use categories of substances. The toxicology is ready to conduct such compound-specific investigations, using biochemical, cellular and tissue culture techniques, including methodologies for measuring gene expression, and last but not least, tailor-made toxicokinetic modelling. I do believe that a drawback of the prominent presence of (OECD-)guidelines for standard tests is negligence of toxicokinetic and mechanism of action studies. Of course, for some widely used chemicals of great commercial interest and with major potential health risks, complex toxicokinetic models have been and are being developed because of the need of very accurate risk estimates. An illustrative example of what can be done is the development of a very sophisticated data- and parameter-rich clonal growth model for formaldehyde by the Chemical Industry Institute of Toxicology (CIIT). The model incorporates over twenty years of research on formaldehyde, and integrates various toxicological, mechanistic and dosimetric data, and greatly reduces the uncertainty levels associated with cancer risk estimates for inhaled formaldehyde (CIIT, 1999).

1.6 Application of Toxicokinetic Data in Hazard Identification

Regulatory agencies and experts committees often shrink back to abandon familiar approaches for hazard identification and risk assessment despite conspicuous scientific shortcomings and clear disadvantages in comparison with newer more sophisticated approaches. Using new methodologies requires courage and a vulnerable disposition, and, most important, the right expertise. One (almost historical) example is the use of body weight (to the power1) versus caloric demand (metabolic rate/body weight to the power 0.75 or 0.67) for scaling up the dose in (small) experimental animals to (large) humans. Although in many cases the use of caloric demand is scientifically more justifiable, body weight (to the power 1) is just routinely still widely used as the basis for dose adjustment. Another example is the use of the benchmark dose (BMD) approach instead of the NOAEL- approach. Although the BMD approach has been shown to be useful and applicable in hazard identification, and indeed helps in getting a more complete picture of the toxicity of a chemical, among other things by dose-response modelling and derivation of critical effect doses for various endpoints, its use in standard setting is still rather limited. Is the BMD approach too complex? Although, indeed it is easier to identify the critical study and the overall NOAEL, and to extrapolate from there, the somewhat greater complexity of this much better and scientifically much sounder approach should not be an excuse not to use it.

In my view the same is true for the use of toxicokinetic models. They may be very complex, and precisely a decade ago we stated in a paper on the extrapolation of animal data to humans: "However, in view of the complexity of these models, it is anticipated that their use will remain restricted", but we also stated: "It should be emphasized that even short-term toxicokinetic data (ADME) including identification of metabolite profiles in test species would certainly make more confident interspecies extrapolation possible" (Feron *et al.*, 1990).

I think, overall, it is the combination of lack of relevant data, the existence of rigid guidelines for toxicity testing, and the reluctance of advisory committees and regulatory agencies to adopt the use of somewhat more complex techniques for hazard identification, which hampers the use of applicable toxicokinetic models in risk assessment. I am convinced that this symposium will contribute significantly to a better insight in the present state of affairs regarding the practical applicability of toxicokinetic models in risk assessment. My conviction is simply based on the presence of so many experienced experts who will discuss various aspects of toxicokinetic models and their applicability and application in risk assessment. I do hope this symposium will stimulate the use of toxicokinetic models in hazard identification and risk assessment. I am sure we will have a very instructive and fruitful meeting, because I believe in the strength of discussion based on facts (data), expertise and experience.

1.7 References

CIIT (1999). Formaldehyde: Hazard and Dose-Response Assessment for Carcinogenicity by the Route of Inhalation; Revised Edition. Chemical Industry Institute of Toxicology, Research Triagle Park.

Feron, V.J. (1998). Recommending health-based exposure limits in the national and international arena: a personal view. In:The Politics of Chemical Risk: Scenarios for a Regulatory Future, Bal, R. and Halffman, W. (Eds.), Kluwer Academic Publishers, Dordrecht, pp.121-129.

Feron, V.J., Hoeksema, C., Arts, J.H.E., Noordam, P.C. and Maas, C.L. (1994). A critical appraisal of setting and implementation of occupational exposure limits in The Netherlands. Indoor Environment, 3, 260-265.

Feron, V.J., van Bladeren, P.J. and Hermus, R.J.J. (1990). A viewpoint on the extrapolation of toxicological data from animals to man. Food and Chemical Toxicology, 28, 783-788.

Munro, I.C., Kennepohl, E. and Kroes, R. (1999), A procedure for the safety evaluation of flavouring substances. Food and Chemical Toxicology, 37, 207-232.

Renwick, A.G. (1989). Pharmacokinetics in toxicology. In: Principles and Methods of Toxicology; Wallace, A. (Ed.), Raven press, New York, pp. 835-878.

2 PHYSIOLOGICALLY BASED PHARMACOKINETIC MODELING OF THE GLYCOL ETHER, 2-BUTOXETHANOL, AND ITS APPLICATION IN HUMAN HEALTH RISK ASSESSMENTS AND EXPOSURE GUIDELINES

RICHARD A. CORLEY

Chemical Dosimetry Group, Pacific NW Nat'l Laboratory, Richland, WA, USA

Abstract: 2-Butoxyethanol (BE), is the most widely used glycol ether solvent with a variety of industrial and consumer applications. BE has, therefore, been the subject of numerous risk assessments and exposure guidelines. Exposure guidelines have been based upon findings of intravascular hemolysis in laboratory animals although it was recognized as early as the 1950's that humans were significantly less sensitive. The species-specificity in hemolysis has prompted numerous investigations into potential mechanisms of action and the relative roles for pharmacokinetics and pharmacodynamics in assessments of human health risk. While the precise mechanism remains elusive, the major metabolite of BE, butoxyacetic acid (BAA), has clearly been shown to be responsible for hemolysis. Thus, the ability to predict the concentrations of BAA in blood as a function of dose, route of exposure and species represents an important opportunity for improving the biological basis in human health risk assessments. To fulfill this need, a physiologically based pharmacokinetic (PBPK) model was developed to simulate the disposition of BE with an emphasis on the kinetics of BAA in blood of rats and humans. This PBPK model was used to determine the hemolytically relevant internal doses of BAA (both maximal blood concentrations [Cmax] and the area under the curve [AUC]) in rats following various toxicity study designs and in humans for a variety of potential oral, dermal and inhalation exposure conditions. The model was used to support a variety of exposure guidelines, including the ECETOC ILV, the ACGIH TLV, and the recent EPA IRIS RfC/RfD. In this manuscript, the circumstances and key research surrounding the development and applications of PBPK modeling to improve the biological basis for human health risk assessments for BE will be reviewed.

2.1 Introduction

Production and uses. 2-Butoxyethanol (BE; ethylene glycol n-butyl ether; EGBE; CAS No. 111-76-2; EINECS No. 203-905-0) is a member of a class of compounds commonly referred to as ethylene glycol ethers. Ethylene glycol ethers are produced by reacting ethylene oxide with various alcohols, including methanol, ethanol, propanol and butanol. As a result of their unique water and organic solubilities, ethylene glycol ethers are often used as co-solvents in both aqueous and solvent-based systems. BE is the most

J. Krüse, H.J.M. Verhaar, and W.K. de Raat (eds.), The Practical Applicability of Toxicokinetic Models in the Risk Assessment of Chemicals, 7-39.

widely used of the ethylene glycol ethers with hundreds of industrial and consumer applications in paints, surface coatings, hard surface cleaners, degreasers and as a feedstock for other chemicals such as butyl glycol acetate and in phthalate and stearate plasticizers (CMA, 1997). In Europe, the total EU production of all butyl glycol ethers is ~181,000 tonnes (CEFIC, 1995). Similar production statistics have been reported for the U.S. (CMA, 1997).

Toxicity. With over 50 years of commercial use, an extensive environmental and toxicological database has been developed for BE. As early as the 1940's, BE was reported to induce hematuria/hemoglobinuria in laboratory animals (Werner *et al.*, 1943a-c). These early findings prompted several researchers to investigate the hemolytic potential of BE in various species and potential mechanisms of action. Carpenter *et al.* (1956) and Tyler (1984) have summarized many of these early research efforts. By the 1950's, it was recognized that humans were relatively resistant to the hemolytic effects of BE and that the major metabolite of BE, butoxyacetic acid (BAA) was likely to be responsible for the observed hemolysis. By the 1980's, a number of studies confirmed that BAA was responsible for hemolysis, the primary response in sensitive species following inhalation, oral or dermal exposures. Additional effects on the liver, kidney, spleen, bone marrow and to a lesser degree, the thymus have been observed but are generally considered to be secondary events related to hemolysis. The weight of evidence indicates that BE is not mutagenic, nor is it a reproductive or developmental toxicant. BE is fetotoxic only at maternally toxic (hemolytic) dose levels. The toxicity of BE has been extensively reviewed by a number of organizations in recent years (e.g. NIOSH, 1990; ECETOC, 1994; Worksafe Australia, 1996; CMA, 1997; WHO, 1998; ATSDR, 1999; EPA, 1999).

The National Toxicology Program (NTP) recently completed two-year rat and mouse inhalation bioassays with BE and have issued a draft report for review by NTP's Board of Scientific Counselors Technical Reports Review Subcommittee (NTP, 1998). In this study, groups of F344/N rats were exposed for 6 hr/d, 5 days/week at 0, 31, 62.5 and 125 ppm while B6C3F1 mice were exposed to 0, 62.5, 125 and 250 ppm BE for up to two years. Nonneoplastic lesions in both sexes of rats included Kupffer cell pigmentation in the livers and hyaline degeneration in the olfactory epithelium. Only the incidence, but not the severity, of the olfactory degeneration was exposure-related and was, therefore, considered an adaptive rather than adverse response. The Kupffer cell pigmentation resulted from hemosiderin deposition secondary to hemolysis. A NOAEL of 31 ppm and a LOAEL of 62.5 ppm was determined for noncancer effects.

In mice, nonneoplastic lesions included forestomach ulcers and epithelial hyperplasia, hematopoietic cell proliferation and hemosiderin pigmentation in the spleen, Kupffer cell pigmentation in the livers, hyaline degeneration of the olfactory epithelium (females only) and bone marrow hyperplasia (males only). As in the rats, the hyaline degeneration in the olfactory epithelium was considered an adaptive response and the Kupffer cell pigmentation in the liver was considered a secondary effect of hemolysis. Bone marrow hyperplasia and hematopoietic cell proliferation and hemosiderin pigmentation in the spleen were also considered secondary to hemolysis with corresponding regeneration in hematopoietic tissues (spleen and bone marrow). The forestomach lesions did not appear to be related to hemolysis and may reflect either a direct irritant effect of BE (oral ingestion due to grooming) or systemic toxicity of BE of its metabolite, BAA. Ongoing research is exploring these hypotheses. A NOAEL could not be determined in mice therefore, the low exposure of 62.5 ppm may be considered a LOAEL for noncancer effects in mice.

For carcinogenic effects in rats, the NTP draft report concluded: "...there was *no evidence of carcinogenic activity* of 2-butoxyethanol in male F344/N rats exposed to 31.2, 62.5 or 125 ppm. There was *equivocal evidence of carcinogenic activity* of 2-butoxyethanol in female F344/N rats based on the increased combined incidences of benign and malignant pheochromocytoma (mainly benign) of the adrenal medula".

The incidence of pheochromocytomas at the highest exposure (16%) was only slightly higher than the upper range of historical controls (13%) and was only marginally significant (p=0.044, trend test). Pheochromocytomas can also be difficult to distinguish from nonneoplastic adrenal medullary hyperplasia and, according to the draft report, these tumors were "small and not substantially larger than the more severe grades of adrenal medullary hyperplasia". Thus, these tumors must be interpreted with caution.

For mice, NTP concluded: "...there was *some evidence of carcinogenic activity* of 2-butoxyethanol in male B6C3F1 mice based on increased incidences of hemangiosarcoma of the liver. A marginal increase in the incidences of forestomach squamous cell papilloma may have been exposure related." NTP also concluded that "There was *some evidence of carcinogenic activity* of 2-butoxyethanol in female B6C3F1 mice based on increased incidences of forestomach squamous cell papilloma or carcinoma (mainly papilloma)".

The hemangiosarcomas in the livers of male mice appeared to be exposure-related. However, the incidence was only slightly higher than historical control ranges (8% vs. 4%), was not increased in other organs and was not noted in female mice or rats. Recent work by Xue *et al.* (1999) suggests that chronic hemolysis and hemosiderin (iron) accumulation in Kupffer cells may lead to increased oxidative stress in the liver. B6C3F1 mice have previously been shown to be more sensitive to oxidative stress than rats or humans (Bachowski *et al.*, 1997). Thus, if the hemangiosarcomas are a result of chronic, hemolysis-induced oxidative stress, then their relevance for human risk is questionable. Ongoing research should help resolve this issue.

The increased incidence of forestomach squamous cell papillomas or carcinomas may have been associated with the chronic toxicity (ulceration and hyperplasia) that was also observed in mice but not in rats. The relevance of forestomach lesions for humans in general, which lack a forestomach, has been the subject of considerable debate. Nevertheless, research is in progress to determine: (a) the potential for oral consumption of BE deposited on the fur of mice following inhalation exposures, (b) whether direct contact with neat BE may lead to forestomach irritation, and (c) whether inhalation exposures leads to preferential accumulation of BE or its metabolites in the forestomachs of mice as has been shown for rats 48 hr after receiving ^{14}C-BE by gavage (Ghanayem *et al.*, 1987b). Since neat BE (vapor of liquid) can be an irritant to the respiratory tract and skin, these additional studies are needed to add perspective to the chronic irritation potential of BE to the forestomach of mice and its potential role in producing a neoplastic response.

2.2 Exposure Guidelines Using Traditional Approaches

When human data are unavailable, occupational exposure limits (OEL) are based upon studies with laboratory animals. In these simple, default calculations, the no-observed effect levels (NOEL) from animal studies are divided by a safety or uncertainty factor to arrive at acceptable 8-hr time-weighted average exposure levels (Eq. 1).

$$\text{OEL} = \text{NOEL}_{\text{animal}} \,/\, \text{Safety or Uncertainty Factor} \quad (1)$$

Generally, the most sensitive sex from the most sensitive species in the most sensitive study is used to define the $\text{NOEL}_{\text{animal}}$. The safety or uncertainty factors are used to compensate for uncertainties associated with the animal toxicity study from which the NOEL is based, uncertainties associated with animal-to-human, high-to-low dose and route-to-route extrapolations, and for potential variability in human response. Under these conditions, there are no formal procedures for incorporating metabolism, pharmacokinetic or mechanistic information. Rather, this information has been used to modify default safety or uncertainty factors as has been done previously with BE.

In 1946 the American Conference of Governmental Industrial Hygienists (ACGIH) established a 200 ppm exposure limit (8-hr time-weighted average) for BE. In 1957, the ACGIH adopted a Threshold Limit Value (TLV) of 50 ppm. In 1964, the ACGIH added a "skin notation" to indicate that precautions should be taken to prevent dermal exposures. In 1981, ACGIH reduced the TLV to 25 ppm. These lower limits were based upon the no-observed effect level (NOEL) for hemolysis observed in a subchronic rat inhalation study (industry-sponsored study published by Dodd *et al.*, in 1983). No additional uncertainty factors were applied to the NOEL since rats were considered to be more sensitive than humans. The German MAK value, also based upon the Dodd *et al.* (1983) study, was set at 20 ppm in 1983. In 1999, ACGIH set the TLV to 20 ppm to be consistent with the German MAK value. Similar exposure limits have been established in other countries and are summarized by ECETOC (1994).

While the ACGIH guidelines are widely used in the U.S., only the Occupational Safety and Health Administration (OSHA) Permissible Exposure Limits are legally enforceable. After its establishment in 1970, OSHA adopted the ACGIH TLV of 50 ppm with a skin notation as the PEL for BE. In 1989, OSHA proposed hundreds of updated PELs, including BE. In 1992, OSHA adopted a PEL of 25 ppm for BE, consistent with the reduced ACGIH TLV. Subsequent litigation overturned all of the newly adopted OSHA limits. As a result, the original 50 ppm PEL remains the current legally enforceable occupational exposure limit in the United States.

When OSHA had proposed a 25 ppm PEL in 1989, the National Institute of Occupational Health (NIOSH) issued a Recommended Exposure Limit (REL) of 5 ppm BE (NIOSH, 1990). While NIOSH agreed that 25 ppm was a NOEL in animals and that humans were less susceptible than animals, it proposed a lower REL to account for potential human variability. Since issuance of this REL, a number of studies have been conducted that have not supported the need for an additional safety factor. The NIOSH REL carries no regulatory authority and neither OSHA nor other more recent governmental reviews have adopted the recommended exposure limit.

For non-occupational exposures in the U.S., the EPA establishes guidelines for continuous, lifetime exposures. These guidelines are documented in their Integrated Risk Information System (IRIS) as reference doses (RfD) for oral exposures and reference concentrations (RfC; formerly referred to as RfD_i or reference dose, inhalation) for inhalation exposures. The oral Reference Dose (RfD) is based on the assumption that thresholds exist for certain toxic effects and is expressed in units of mg/kg/day. As defined by the EPA, an RfD is an estimate (with uncertainty spanning perhaps an order of magnitude) of a daily exposure to the human population, including sensitive subpopulations, that is likely to be without an appreciable risk of deleterious effects during a lifetime. The inhalation RfC, expressed in units of mg/m^3, is analogous to the RfD, but also considers toxic effects for the respiratory system (portal of entry effects).

In 1991, the IRIS group developed a RfC for continuous, lifetime inhalation exposures to BE, although it was not finalized and added to the IRIS database pending EPA's evaluation of new data being developed on the toxicity, mode of action and dosimetry of BE. However, the 'provisional' RfC of 0.02 mg/m^3 (4 ppb) was published in HEAST tables. As with other contemporary occupational exposure guidelines, the provisional RfC was based upon the subchronic rat inhalation study of Dodd *et al.* (1983) according to the following calculations:

$$\text{RfC (mg/m}^3) = \text{OAEL*}_{[HEC]} / (\text{UF x MF}) = (22\ \text{mg/m}^3)/(1000 * 1) = 0.02\ \text{mg/m}^3 \quad (2)$$

where:

$$\text{NOAEL*}_{[HEC]} = \text{NOAEL*}_{[ADJ]}\ (\text{mg/m}^3) \times \lambda_{blood:air}\ \text{animal}/\lambda_{blood:air}\ \text{human} = (22\ \text{mg/m}^3) * 1 = 22\ \text{mg/m}^3 \quad (3)$$

and:

$$\text{NOAEL*}_{[ADJ]} = \text{NOAEL (mg/m}^3) * \text{no. hr exposed/24 hr} * \text{no. days exposed per week/7 days per week} \quad (4)$$
$$= (121\ \text{mg/m}^3) * 6/24 * 5/7 = 22\ \text{mg/m}^3$$

The NOEL of 25 ppm from the Dodd *et al.* (1983) study was used as the animal NOAEL after converting the units to 121 mg/m^3. The animal NOAEL was adjusted for a continuous human exposure assuming Haber's Law of concentration x time was appropriate. Thus, the adjusted NOAEL ($\text{NOAEL*}_{[ADJ]}$) was calculated in Eq. 4 to convert from a 6 hr/day, 5 day/week exposure regimen. The human equivalent concentration NOAEL ($\text{NOAEL*}_{[HEC]}$) was then calculated according to Eq. 3 by multiplying the adjusted NOAEL by the ratio of animal to human blood:air partition coefficients. Since these values were unknown for BE, a default value of 1 for the ratio was used in this equation. An overall uncertainty factor (UF) of 1000 and a modifying factor of 1 was then used in Eq. 2 to arrive at the provisional RfC. The overall UF of 1000 reflected uncertainty factors of 10 for animal to human extrapolation, 10 to protect sensitive humans and 10 to extrapolate from subchronic to chronic exposures and the limited reproductive information available for BE at the time the calculation was made.

In the 1990's, this provisional RfC, available in HEAST tables, was often cited inappropriately and used by several organizations, government and otherwise, to establish occupational and chronic exposure guidelines. The provisional RfC was, at the time, the lowest RfC (provisional or otherwise) assigned by the EPA for any glycol ether. Contrary to what this provisional RfC suggested, BE appeared to be one of the least toxic of the ethylene glycol ethers to humans. This contributed to the confusion over the relative risks of exposure to glycol ethers during a period of intense scrutiny over the use of structurally similar developmentally and reproductively toxic glycol ethers.

2.3 Rationale for the Development of a PBPK Model for BE

By the late 1980's a combination of issues, regulatory activities and scientific research set the stage for the development of a PBPK model for BE that could be used to improve the scientific basis for human health risk assessments (summarized in Table 1). While early research clearly indicated that BE's toxicity was unique among structurally similar glycol ethers, the finding that ME and EE, when metabolized to their corresponding alkoxyacetic acid, could affect the bone marrow, testes or developing fetus in laboratory animals was causing agencies around the world to carefully scrutinize all glycol ethers for potential risks to human health. In the past, this has led to varying degrees of confusion on the part of many authorities involved in the classification or establishment of exposure guidelines whenever the distinctive toxicological characteristics of these otherwise structurally similar chemicals were not appreciated.

With BE representing one of the highest production volume glycol ethers with a variety of industrial and consumer applications, there was considerable interest by a number of groups to follow up on decades of research on species-differences in toxicity to understand the relevance of animal studies for human exposures. In the late 1980's, the National Toxicology Program (NTP) conducted a series of studies on the metabolism and modes of action of BE in preparation for chronic toxicity/oncogenicity testing. As a part of this program, Ghanayem *et al.* published a series of papers demonstrating that the BE-induced hemolysis was directly attributable to the formation of the BAA from BE via alcohol and aldehyde dehydrogenases (Ghanayem *et al.*, 1987a and b; Ghanayem, 1989; Ghanayem *et al.*, 1990). In addition, they found that human red blood cells were significantly less sensitive than red blood cells from rats when incubated directly with BAA *in vitro*. However, Dr. Ghanayem also hypothesized that there may potentially be sensitive subpopulations of people predisposed to hemolytic anemia by certain disorders such as hereditary spherocytosis, glucose-6-phosphate dehydrogenase deficiency and sickle cell anemia which could be at a higher risk than healthy humans (Ghanayem, 1989). Furthermore, Ghanayem postulated that the elderly could be at greater risk since BE-induced hemolysis was age-dependent in rats and several potentially important biochemical defense mechanisms

Table 1. Driving forces behind the development of a PBPK model for 2-butoxyethanol and 2-butoxyacetic acid.

- Unwarranted categorical classifications of structurally similar ethylene glycol ethers by regulatory authorities despite significant differences in toxicity observed between BE and other members of its chemical class.
- Numerous authorities were re-evaluating BE health risks and proposing new exposure guidelines based upon default procedures and uncertainty factors.
- The HEAST value (provisional RfC) of 0.02 mg/m^3 (4 ppb) for continuous, lifetime exposure was being inappropriately cited and used by state and local authorities to establish occupational exposure guidelines.
- The cancer risk assessment for methylene chloride was impacted by PBPK modeling setting a precedent for further use of PBPK models.
- The U.S.E.P.A. recommended the use of PBPK models in non-cancer, reference concentration/reference dose calculations.
- Analytical methods for analysis of BE and eventually BAA in blood were developed which allowed the conduct of numerous kinetic studies in rats and humans following several routes of exposure.
- A human PBPK model for BE inhalation exposure was published by Johanson in 1986.
- The U.S. National Toxicology Program initiated a series of metabolism, mode of action and subchronic studies as a prelude to the design of chronic bioassays with glycol ethers.
- The metabolism of BE to BAA was hypothesized by Carpenter (1956) and later demonstrated by Ghanayem *et al.* (1987) to be a requirement for hemolysis.
- Rat blood was shown *in vitro* to be more sensitive than normal human blood to BAA-induced hemolysis; speculations were raised by Ghanayem (1990) regarding potentially susceptible human subpopulations.

Additional mechanism studies and *in vitro* comparisons between rat and human blood and blood from individuals potentially predisposed to hemolytic anemia were in progress; relevance to realistic *in vivo* exposures not well-established.

are reportedly compromised in aged animals and humans (Ghanayem, 1989; Ghanayem *et al.* 1990).

As a result of Ghanayem's research findings, the Chemical Manufacturers Association Ethylene Glycol Ethers (CMA-EGE) Panel embarked upon a new research program in 1989 with Dr. Mark Udden, a clinical hematologist at the Baylor College of Medicine. Dr. Udden's research focused on three main areas including: (1) a comparison of BAA-induced hemolytic sensitivity between red blood cells from humans vs. rats, (2) evaluation of hemolysis in blood from potentially susceptible human subpopulations and (3) determination of the mechanism(s) behind the species differences in hemolysis.

Since the species comparisons were to be conducted in vitro, it was critical to understand whether or not realistic environmental exposures to BE would lead to blood concentrations of BAA that produced hemolysis in vitro, especially if it was determined that humans with blood disorders were predisposed to hemolysis. It was becoming widely recognized at that time that physiologically based pharmacokinetic (PBPK) models were well-suited for deriving estimates of tissue doses as a function of administered dose or exposure, route of administration, or species. Furthermore, the utility of PBPK modeling in risk assessment had been established with the employment of the Andersen *et al.* (1987) PBPK model by Canada and the U.S. in their re-evaluations of methylene chloride's carcinogenic risk. Therefore, the development and validation of a rat and human PBPK model was considered an integral component in the CMA-EGE Panel's overall research program.

Additional incentive for model development was provided in 1990 by the EPA when they released for external review and comments, a draft of their interim guidance document recommending the use of validated PBPK models to replace default procedures in determining non-cancer, reference concentrations (RfC) for continuous lifetime exposures to chemicals. This draft interim guidance document, which was finalized in 1994, represented the first formal process by a regulatory agency for incorporating biologically motivated mechanistic and dosimetric information, such as a PBPK model, into exposure guidelines for human health risk assessments (EPA, 1994). This new approach, coupled with the willingness of EPA scientists to work collaboratively with industrial, academic and government researchers, provided significant motivation for industry to continue sponsoring this line of research in general, as well as for BE specifically.

2.4 Development of a Rat and Human PBPK model for BE and BAA

In 1990, the CMA-EGE Panel initiated several research studies that led to the development and validation of a multi-route, rat and human PBPK model for BE and it's hemolytic metabolite, BAA (Corley *et al.* in 1994; Bormett *et al.*, 1995; Markham *et al.*, 1995; Corley *et al.*, 1997). This model was structured around the Johanson (1986) human PBPK model for BE. Several of the leading researchers on the metabolism and kinetics of BE including Drs. Johanson, Ghanayem and Sabourin, made significant contributions to the design or conduct of many of the studies. During the course of model development, Shyr *et al.* (1993) published a rat PBPK model designed to describe data from their laboratory's pharmacokinetic studies of BE administered by drinking water, inhalation and dermal routes of exposure. In 1998, Lee *et al.* updated the CMA-sponsored PBPK model to simulate the data from the NTP pharmacokinetic study conducted in parallel with their chronic rat and mouse inhalation bioassays. Both the Corley *et al.* (1994 and 1997) and Lee *et al.* (1998) models were used by the EPA to develop the RfC and RfD for BE. Each of these models is briefly described below.

Johanson (1986) human inhalation PBPK model. The original PBPK model of Johanson (1986), which formed the basis for all subsequent models, was developed to describe the concentration of unmetabolized BE in the blood of humans exposed to 20 ppm BE vapor for 2 hr while exercising (data from Johanson *et al.*, 1986a). The structure of Johanson's model was similar to other contemporary blood flow-limited models of organic solvents. Johanson assumed that the uptake of BE during the exposure occurred only via the lungs and metabolism (elimination of BE) occurred only in the liver, thus these two compartments were also explicitly defined. The gastrointestinal tract and fat compartments were also explicitly defined as they were for other organic solvents. The muscle and skin were separated from the slowly perfused tissue compartment because of their differential blood flows during exercise. Other tissues that were not important for either the uptake or metabolism of BE were combined into one of two compartments depending on their relative blood perfusion rates. BE was assumed to distribute instantaneously within each compartment (also known as a well-stirred compartment). Thus, the concentration in any non-metabolic tissue was driven by the tissue:blood partition coefficient and the blood flow to that tissue. A schematic of Johanson's PBPK model for BE is shown in Figure 1.

The blood:air partition coefficient of 7965 for BE was determined by vial equilibration (Johanson and Dynesius, 1988). All tissue:blood partition coefficients were not measured but were assumed to be unity. Consistent with other water soluble organic chemicals, the relative pulmonary uptake was set to 60% of the alveolar ventilation rate based on the kinetic data of Johanson *et al.* (1986a). The metabolism of BE, via alcohol and aldehyde dehydrogenases, in the liver was described by a single, saturable, Michaelis-Menten kinetic equation. Metabolic rate constants were determined from perfused rat

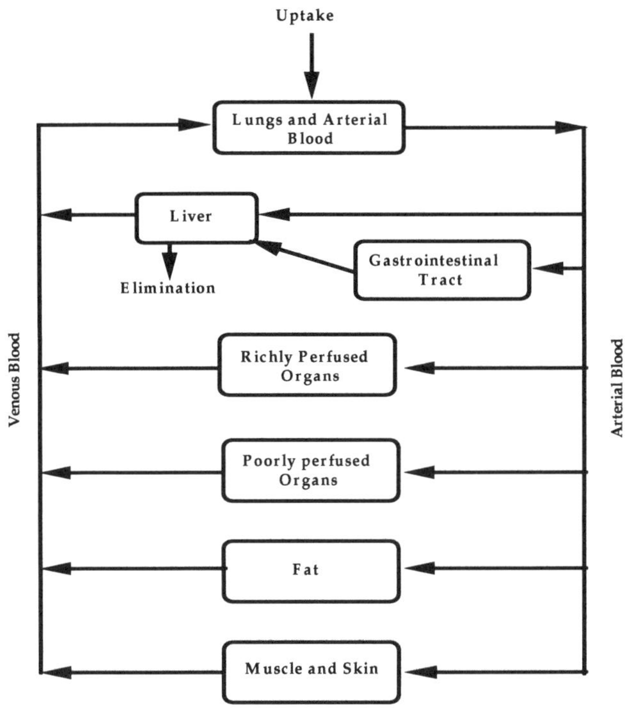

Figure 1. Diagramatic representation of the PBPK model for 2-butoxyethanol kinetics in humans exposed by inhalation (from Johanson, 1986).

liver experiments (Johanson *et al.*, 1986b). The human metabolic capacity (Vmax) was scaled from the rat to the human by the (body weight)$^{0.74}$.

While Johanson's model adequately described the kinetics of BE in the blood of humans exposed via inhalation, no attempts were made at that time to analyze for, or simulate the kinetics of the hemolytic metabolitc, BAA, in blood. Five years after conducting the human kinetic study, analytical methods were developed and several blood and urine samples from the human kinetic study were analyzed for BAA and reported by Johanson and Johnsson (1991). An average peak blood concentration of 44 μM BAA (range: 36 - 57 μM) was reached 2-4 hr post-exposure. The average $t_{1/2}$ for elimination of BAA from blood was 4.3 hr (range: 1.7 - 9.6 hr) suggesting little chance of accumulation of BAA following repeated occupational exposures to concentrations at or below existing occupational exposure limits of 20 - 25 ppm. The average renal clearance of BAA was 23-39 ml/min, which was only about one-third of the glomerular filtration rate. Johanson and Johnsson suggested that the low clearance of BAA relative to the glomerular filtration rate could have been related to the binding of BAA to proteins in blood or to a low efficiency in renal tubular secretion. The low pKa of 3.5 (estimated by Johanson and Johnsson) indicated that tubular reabsorption was unlikely since more than 99% of the BAA in normal human urine (pH ~6) is ionized. The volume of distribution (Vd) averaged 15 L (range: 6.5 - 25 L), based on whole blood measurements, which was approximately equal to the volume of extracellular water (13-16 L), a further indication of binding of BAA to blood proteins. These data were not used by Johanson and Johnsson to expand their PBPK model to include a description of BAA in blood but were used by Corley *et al.* (1994 and 1997).

Shyr et al. (1993) multi-route rat PBPK model. Shyr *et al.* (1993) developed a PBPK model to describe data collected in their laboratory on the metabolism of BE in F344 rats following dermal (Sabourin *et al.*, 1992b), drinking water (Medinsky *et al.*, 1990) or nose-only inhalation (Sabourin *et al.*, 1992a) exposures. The model structure for BE was based on the Johanson (1986) model and included the respiratory tract, liver, GI tract, fat, skin, muscle and richly perfused tissues (Figure 2). The model incorporated metabolism of BE in the liver to either: (a) BAA via alcohol/aldehyde dehydrogenases, (b) ethylene glycol (EG) via mixed function oxidase, or (c) reversible conjugation with glucuronic acid. In addition, glucuronide conjugation was also assumed to occur in the skin to successfully simulate data from the dermal exposure study.

The metabolic parameters for the formation of BAA, EG and glucuronide conjugate of BE were assumed to follow Michaelis-Menten kinetics with a Km and Vmax to describe the affinity and capacity, respectively for each pathway. Estimates of these parameters were obtained by fitting the data from the three metabolism studies with the constraint that the sum of the individual metabolic rates for each pathway was similar to the value for total

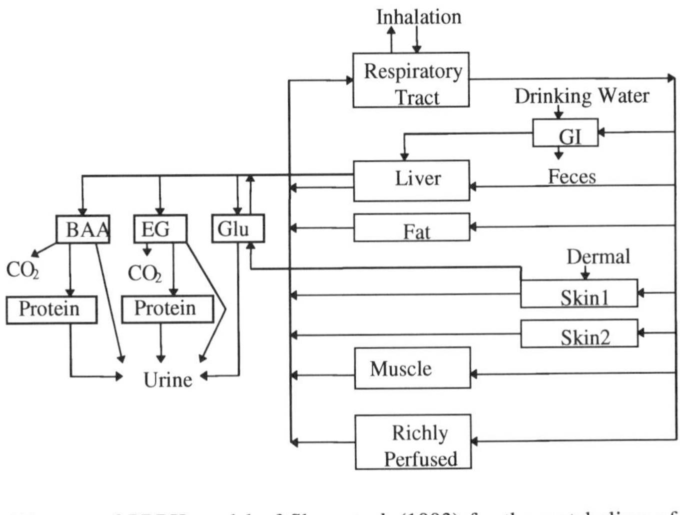

Figure 2. Diagram of PBPK model of Shyr *et al.* (1993) for the metabolism of BE in rats following drinking water, inhalation and dermal exposure. Skin1 is the volume on which the dermal dose was applied and Skin2 was the remainder of the skin compartment.

metabolism derived by Johanson *et al.* (1986b) using isolated, perfused rat livers. Partition coefficients for BE were assumed to be 0.9 (based on the ratio of the water:air partition coefficient of 7051 to the blood:air coefficient of 7965 as measured by Johanson and Dynesius (1988)) for all tissues except the fat, which was set to 0.7 (based on using the oil:air partition coefficient 5446 as a surrogate). A sensitivity analysis by Shyr *et al.*, indicated that the parameters that had the most impact on model simulations included the metabolic rate constants for the formation of the various metabolites and the blood flow to the liver. No attempts were made to fit the data from other rat metabolism studies to independently validate the parameters used in their model. However, Corley *et al.* (1994) successfully modeled these and other data sets with a similar model structure (except metabolic pathways leading to EG and glucuronide conjugates were combined) indicating that many of the parameters used by Shyr *et al.*, were reasonable. As with the original Johanson (1986) model, no attempts were made to collect data or to simulate the concentration of BAA in blood, thus, limiting its use in risk assessment.

Corley et al. (1994 and 1997) PBPK model for BE and BAA. The main objective of the CMA-EGE Panel-sponsored program was to upgrade the Johanson (1986) PBPK model to describe the concentration of BAA in the target tissue (blood) of rats and humans as an internal dose surrogate for assessing the potential risk for hemolysis. Several modifications were made to Johanson's model to accomplish this objective. Standard (fixed) physiological and biochemical parameters for a 70-kg human were converted to allometrically scalable parameters adjustable by the actual body weights of the subjects in several human kinetic studies. The physiology of humans under exercise conditions was maintained in the model in addition to the physiology at rest. The rat was included to provide an interspecies comparison of target tissue doses (BAA in blood) in risk assessments and to expand the database for model validation. To make use of a variety of published studies, the Corley *et al.* (1994) model included additional routes of exposure such as oral gavage, drinking water, dermal (liquids and vapor) and intravenous infusion. To model dermal exposures to either liquids or vapor, the combined muscle and skin compartment of Johanson's model was separated into individual components. The formation of BAA was assumed to occur only in the liver using the rat liver perfusion data of Johanson *et al.* (1986b) scaled to the human. A second model was linked to the BE model specifically to track the disposition of BAA, following its formation in the liver. The kidney was added to the BAA model since it is the primary organ of elimination for BAA. All other metabolic routes for BE (formation of EG and glucuronide conjugates) that were specified in the Shyr *et al.* (1993) model were combined since they were only used to account for the total disposition of BE in the rat metabolism studies and not for cross-species extrapolations. The PBPK model structure is shown in Figure 3.

Partition coefficients for both BE and BAA were measured in human blood, rat blood and rat tissues. Human tissue:blood partition coefficients were assumed to be equal to the rat. For most tissues, the measured partition coefficients validated the assumption of Johanson (1986) that BE would have relatively equivalent solubility in tissues versus blood. According to a sensitivity analysis, even those tissues partition coefficients which deviated significantly from unity had little impact on model output (Lee *et al.*, 1995). Thus, the slight differences in partition coefficients used by each of the published PBPK models are considered to be insignificant. As alluded to by Johanson and Johnsson (1991), protein binding of BAA in blood and saturable elimination of BAA by the kidneys were also necessary components to describe the BAA kinetic data in rats and humans.

Several rat metabolism studies were simulated with the PBPK model of Corley *et al.* (1994). These simulations included data from rats administered BE by intravenous infusion (Ghanayem *et al.*, 1990) and oral gavage (Ghanayem *et al.*, 1987a,b). Consistent with the Shyr *et al.* (1993) model,

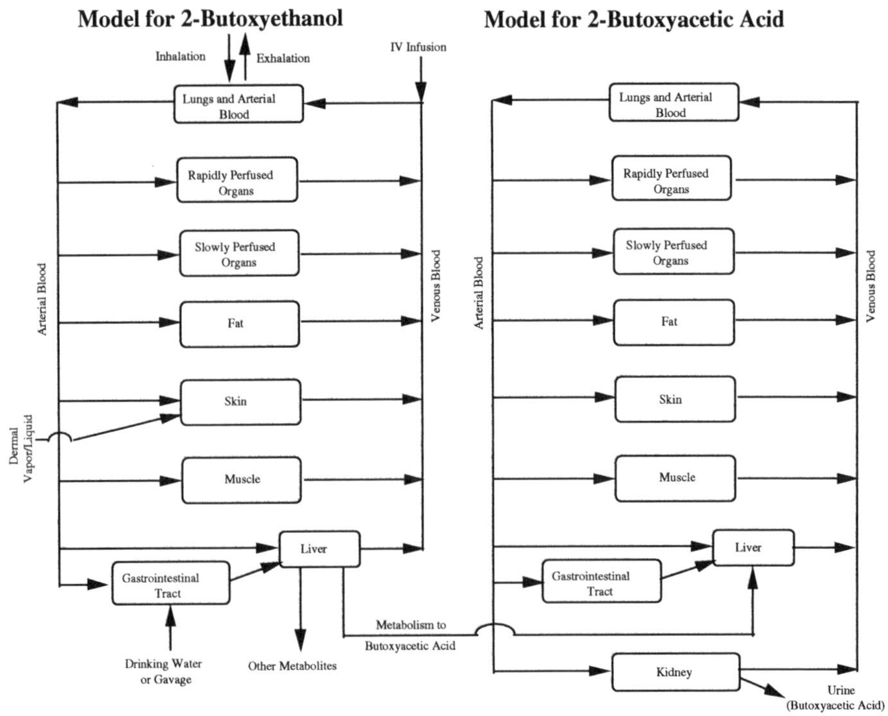

Figure 3. PBPK model of Corley *et al.* (1994). The formation of BAA from BE was assumed to occur only in the liver and was simulated in a second model linked via the formation of BAA.

this model also simulated the amounts of BAA and other metabolites (totals only) eliminated in the urine from rats following drinking water (Medinsky *et al.*, 1990) and nose-only inhalation exposures (Sabourin *et al.*, 1992). An additional oral kinetic study was conducted by Corley *et al.* (1994) to validate the model's ability to simulate the concentration of BAA in the blood of rats. This study was necessary since the only other BE and BAA blood concentration data that was available at the time (Ghanayem *et al.*, 1990) was used to determine rate constants for renal elimination of BAA. To conduct this, and subsequent human kinetic studies, new gas chromatography/mass spectrometry analytical methods having the sensitivity and selectivity to simultaneously quantitate BE and BAA at either very low (ppb) levels using very small sample volumes (0.1 ml) were developed (Bormett *et al.*, 1995).

The Corley *et al.* (1994) model also adequately described human data from several studies. These studies included the Johanson *et al.* (1986a) human exposure to 20 ppm BE during exercise and the Johanson and Johnsson (1991) subsequent analysis of BAA in blood. In addition, Johanson and Boman (1991) attempted to define the relative importance of the skin to the total absorption of BE vapor in whole-body exposures and concluded that dermal uptake was appreciably higher (~3-fold) than respiratory uptake. This study impacted ongoing efforts to establish exposure guidelines since its conclusions indicated that respiratory protection might not be adequate. Thus, additional research was necessary.

In the Johanson and Boman (1991) study, human volunteers were exposed to 50 ppm BE vapor using the following regimen: two hr of mouth-only exposure followed by one hr of no exposure followed by two hr of body only exposure (dressed in shorts only, fresh breathing air supplied by a respirator). Each subject showered immediately after the body-only exposure. The experiment was replicated at normal and raised temperatures and humidities. Finger-prick blood samples were collected periodically for analysis of BE. Assuming that the finger prick blood sample technique used by Johanson and Boman represented venous blood draining the skin prior to mixing systemically and not mixed arterial blood, provided the most consistent simulation of all available human data (Corley *et al.*, 1994). These simulations were confirmed in a follow-up human kinetic study (Corley *et al.*, 1997).

In the Corley *et al.* (1997) study, human volunteers exposed one arm only to 50 ppm ^{13}C-BE for 2 hr. Catheters installed in the antecubital vein of the unexposed arm served as the primary site for blood collection and analyzed for both BE and BAA. Finger prick blood samples were collected from the exposed arm at the end of the two-hr exposure according to the methods of Johanson and Boman (1991). Urine was collected for 24 hr for identification and quantitation of metabolites. These data and PBPK simulations of human skin permeability indicated that respiratory absorption of BE vapor in a whole-body exposure was at least 3-6 fold (under worst-case conditions) to as much as 10 or even 100-fold more important under more realistic exposure scenarios than dermal absorption. In addition, the elimination kinetics of BE and BAA in this study were consistent with previous studies by Johanson *et al.* and appeared to be independent of the route of exposure. The half-lives for the elimination of BE and BAA averaged 0.66 hr and 3.27 hr, respectively. For whole-body exposures under exercise conditions, the elimination half-lives for BE and BAA were 0.66 and 4 hr, respectively (Johanson *et al.*, 1986a; Johanson and Johnsson, 1991). For dermal exposure to neat liquids, the half-lives for elimination of BE and BAA were 1.3 hr and 3.1 hr, respectively (Johanson *et al.*, 1988). For dermal exposure to vapors, the elimination half-life for BE was 0.53-0.6 hr.

Contrary to observations in rats, Corley *et al.* (1997) also found no evidence of metabolites in urine that would indicate that humans formed ethylene glycol or conjugates of BE. Thus, these pathways, which were combined in the model of Corley *et al.* (1994) to simulate rat kinetic data, were eliminated for human simulations. This study also confirmed the observations of Rettenmeier *et al.* (1993) that approximately two-thirds of the BAA formed by humans is conjugated with glutamine and to a lesser extent, glycine. This is a pathway that has not been detected in the rat. Simulations of all of the human kinetic data using the revised model of Corley *et al.* (1997) are shown in Figures 4 and 5.

(a)

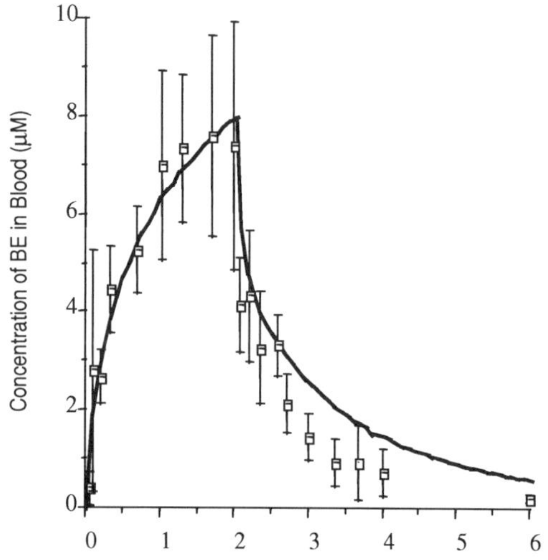

Figure 4a. Comparison between experimental data and simulations of the concentrations of BE in the blood of humans exposed either (a) whole-body for 2 hr to 20 ppm BE while exercising (Johanson *et al.*, 1986b) … (b) and c) continued on next page).

(b)

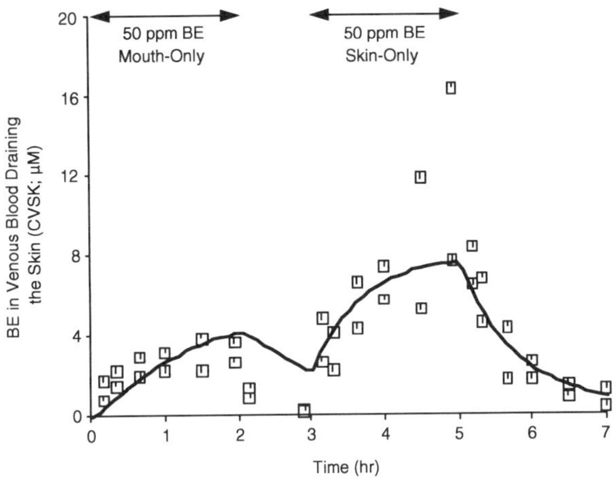

(c)

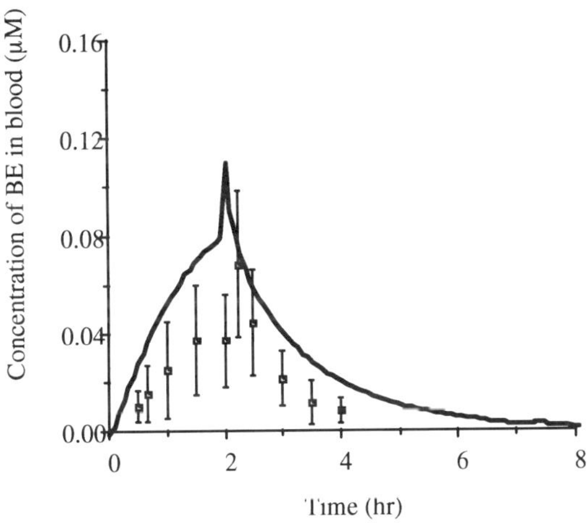

Figure 4. Comparison between experimental data and simulations of the concentrations of BE in the blood of humans exposed either (a) whole-body for 2 hr to 20 ppm BE while exercising (Johanson *et al.*, 1986b) (previous page); (b) mouth-only for 2hr to 50 ppm BE followed by one hr of no exposure followed by 2 hr of body-only exposure to 50 ppm BE (Johanson and Boman, 1991); and (c) arm-only to 50 ppm ^{13}C-BE for 2 hr (Corley *et al.*, 1997).

(a)

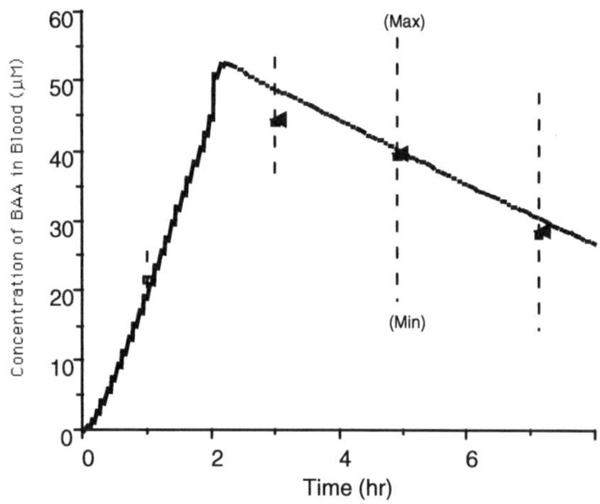

(b)

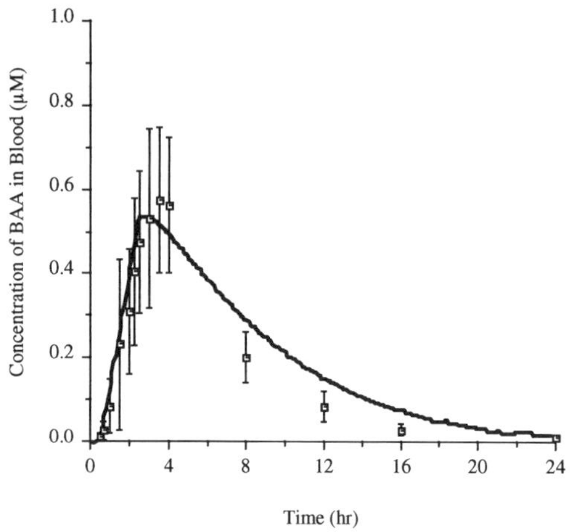

Figure 5. Comparison between experimental data and simulations of the concentrations of BAA in the blood of humans exposed (a) whole-body for 2 hr to 20 ppm BE while exercising (Johanson and Johnsson, 1991) and (b) arm-only to 50 ppm 13C-BE for 2 hr (from Corley *et al.*, 1997).

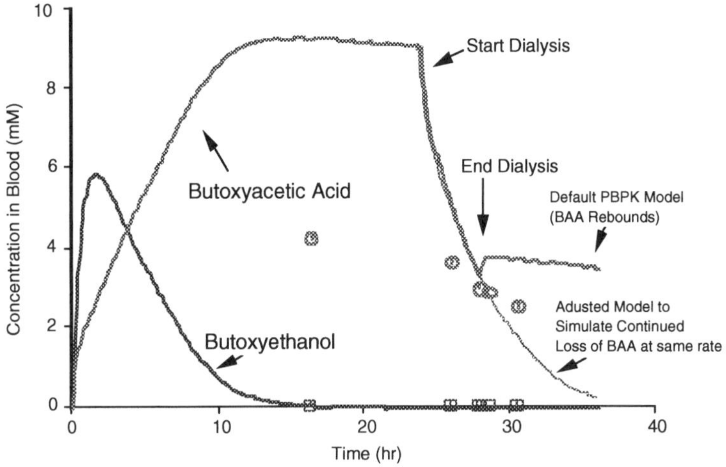

Figure 6. Concentrations of BE and BAA (symbols) in the blood of a 71 kg male following an intentional ingestion of 360-480 ml of a concentrated window cleaner containing 22% BE. Simulations (lines) conducted with Corley *et al.* (1997) PBPK model.

The ability of the PBPK model to adequately simulate high-dose human exposures to BE was demonstrated by Gualtieri *et al.* (1995) in a case report of an intentional suicide attempt with an industrial-strength window cleaner. An 18 year-old 71 kg male consumed between 360-480 ml of a concentrated glass cleaner containing 22% BE. The patient was admitted to the hospital within 3 hr post-ingestion with no abnormalities other than epigastric discomfort. Approximately 10 hr post-admission, the patient was noticeably more lethargic, weak and hyperventilating, consistent with the onset of metabolic acidosis. The patient was transferred to a tertiary care hospital where hemodialysis was initiated (approximately 24 hr post-ingestion) and ethanol therapy was started 30 minutes later. Treatment also consisted of intravenous doses of 100 mg thiamine and 50 mg folic acid every 12 hr, and 50 mg pyridoxine every 6 hr. Following 4 hr of dialysis, the patient was alert and remained hemodynamically stable. Several serum samples were analyzed for BE and BAA and are shown in Figure 6 along with model simulations assuming a total dose of 80 g of BE (1.13 g/kg body weight) was ingested.

Ingestion, ethanol thereapy did have an impact on the disposition of BE (higher concentrations were detected than following the first ingestion) and BAA (lower levels were detected). As with the first episode, clinical manifestations of high dose oral ingestion of nearly 1.1-1.5 g/kg body weight consisted of metabolic acidosis. No evidence of hemolysis was detected.

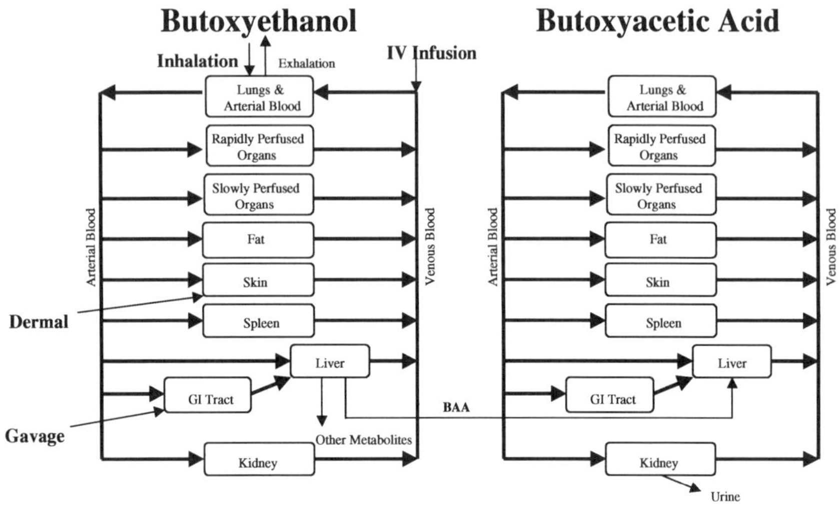

Figure 7. PBPK model of Lee *et al.* (1998). The formation of BAA from BE was assumed to occur only in the liver and was simulated in a second model linked via the formation of BAA.

Lee et al. (1998) rat and mouse inhalation PBPK model. Lee *et al.* (1998) developed a PBPK model to describe the pharmacokinetics of BE and BAA in rats and mice chronically exposed to BE in the NTP bioassay (Dill *et al.*, 1998). When Lee *et al.* tried to simulate the male rat kinetic data from Dill *et al.* (1998) using the Corley *et al.* (1994) male rat model parameters, the model substantially underpredicted both the blood concentration and urinary elimination of BAA. Lee *et al.* attributed this underprediction to either the limited BE uptake or lower rates of metabolism of BE to BAA used by Corley *et al.* to describe data from male rats. The authors therefore, substantially re-structured the Corley *et al.* (1994) model to focus on describing the NTP data and included parameters for female rats and male and female mice as a function of age and chronic exposure.

The muscle compartment was combined with the slowly perfused tissue groups and a spleen compartment was added to both the BE and BAA submodels. A kidney compartment was also added to the BE submodel. Lee *et al.* modified the physiological compartments using slightly different allometric equations to describe tissue volumes as a function of body weight (from Mordenti, 1986) and re-optimized or adjusted several model parameters, including the Km for metabolism of BE to BAA and the number of protein binding sites in plasma (P, mg/liter) to fit the NTP data. Equations for the growth of the animals during the chronic study as a function of gender, species and exposure concentration were described using second- or third-order polynomials fit to the Dill *et al.* (1998) body weight data. Time-dependent changes in cardiac output and volume of the fat were included. Time-dependent chemical parameters, such as the enzyme capacity for BAA formation (male rats only), renal elimination and protein binding were also adjusted to improve the fit the chronic kinetic data. Lee *et al.* maintained the three distinct metabolism pathways for BE from the Shyr *et al.* (1993) model. A diagram of the Lee *et al.* (1998) model is shown in Figure 7.

Many of the changes in physiology used to describe the relative differences in the kinetics of BE and BAA in male and female rats and mice over the course of chronic exposures were supported by numerous independent citations. In fact, additional research sponsored by the CMA-EGE Panel substantiated many of the hypotheses of Lee *et al.* for the age, sex and species differences in metabolism, protein binding and renal elimination (Grant *et al.* 1997; Grant *et al.*, 1998; Farris, 1998) and revisions to the chronic PBPK model are planned. However, the absolute concentrations of BAA in the initial male rat kinetic data set of Dill *et al.* (1998) following either a single exposure or 2 weeks of exposure are significantly higher than expected from other kinetic studies in male rats, the only sex and species of laboratory animals where kinetic data were available for comparison. Thus, changing model parameters to fit these higher concentrations resulted in less optimal simulations (overestimations of BAA concentrations in blood) of other available literature data from male rats used by Corley *et al.* (1994) to develop their model, including a subsequent male rat inhalation kinetic study reported by Johanson (1994). The reason for differences between the Dill *et al.* (1998) data on male rats and other data sets are unknown.

As described below, EPA considered the NTP inhalation toxicity study, with female rats being the most sensitive sex and species for hemolytic effects, as the principle study for determination of the inhalation RfC. Therefore, the Lee *et al.* (1998) model was used to calculate steady-state internal dose estimates of BAA in blood for female rats for RfC calculations while the Corley *et al.* (1994) and (1997) models were used in RfD calculations and in calculations of human equivalent concentrations for both the RfC and RfD.

2.5 Use of PBPK model in Risk Assessments

Species comparisons of target tissue doses. Two potential internal dose surrogates were proposed by Corley *et al.* (1994), each with advantages and disadvantages. The peak blood concentration, Cmax, of BAA is one potential internal dose relevant to hemolysis. Cmax has the advantage in that it is sensitive to dose-rate (e.g. higher Cmax's are achieved following bolus oral dosing than an equivalent dose provided over time via drinking water) however, it is difficult to verify model predictions without adequate numbers of blood samples. In addition, using Cmax for BAA in blood as the internal dose surrogate for hemolysis implies that hemolysis is an instantaneous process, which is unlikely. The alternative internal dose surrogate, area under the curve (AUC) for BAA in blood, integrates the toxicokinetics of BAA over time. However, this internal dose surrogate is not dose-rate sensitive (e.g. the same AUC for BAA is achieved following either a single bolus oral dose or the same dose via the drinking water at dose levels below metabolic saturation).

A comparison of simulated peak blood concentrations for BAA in rats and humans exposed for 6 hr to varying concentrations of BE in the air is presented in Figure 9. Assuming a direct correlation exists between the peak blood concentration and hemolysis in *in vitro* experiments (Figure 9), the Corley *et al.* (1994) model would predict that airborne concentrations >200 ppm would produce significant and potentially lethal hemolysis in rats (Cmax BAA > 0.5 mM). This is consistent with the *in vivo* acute toxicity of Sabourin *et al.*, (1992a) and Tyler (1984). The Lee *et al.* (1998) model predicted similar blood Cmax's of BAA (0.5 mM) following exposures of female rats to ~62 ppm BE. In contrast, peak blood concentrations of BAA in humans will not reach concentrations causing pre-hemolytic changes *in vitro* (8 mM; Ghanayem, 1989; Udden, 1995) even at saturated atmospheric concentrations.

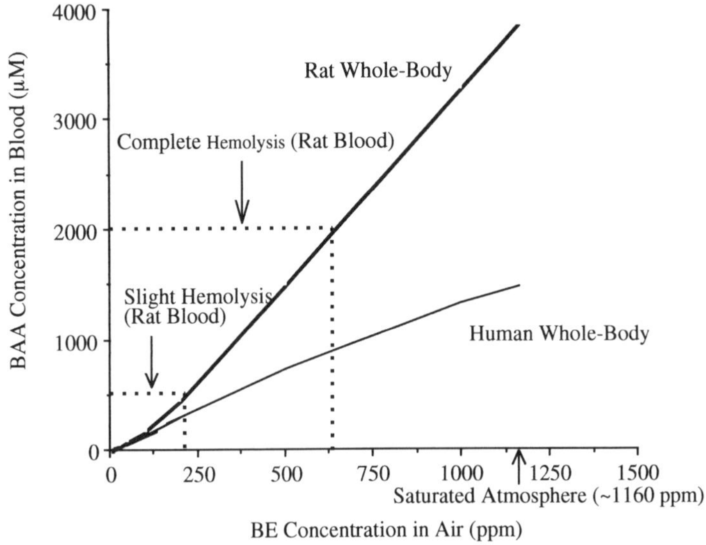

Figure 9. Simulations of peak concentrations (Cmax) for BAA in the blood of rats and humans exposed for 6 hr to various concentrations of BE in air. Simulations were conducted for whole-body exposures (including dermal uptake) and, for humans, no clothing that would hinder dermal absorption using the Corley *et al.* (1997) model.

Impact of PBPK modeling on occupational exposure limits. Both the recent ACGIH (1999) and ECETOC (1994) guidance documents used the PBPK model of Corley *et al.* (1994) as an aid in establishing an exposure limit of 20 ppm for an 8-hr TWA, based upon the Dodd *et al.* (1983) subchronic rat inhalation study. ECETOC relied on a comparison of AUC's and Cmax's for the concentration of BAA in blood of rats and humans to eliminate the interspecies assessment factor and the need for a route of exposure factor (e.g. account for dermal absorption of vapors). PBPK modeling demonstrated adequate margins of safety for humans exposed at the proposed ILV (e.g. Cmax for BAA in blood of humans were several hundred-fold lower than levels likely to cause pre-hemolytic changes). A similar rationale was used to substantiate the lack of a need for additional safety factors for the ACGIH TLV.

Establishment of an EPA RfC and RfD. Following EPA's 1990 release of their draft guidance document for the development of RfC's, the CMA-EGE Panel fostered interactions between researchers involved in the CMA and NTP-sponsored programs and EPA scientists involved in the development of RfC methodologies. The purpose of these interactions was to discuss new research with BE and the potential impact it would have on the development of a new RfC for BE to replace the provisional RfC in the HEAST tables. Discussions also focused on the identification of potential data gaps or areas of concern that could have an impact on establishment of a RfC. Areas identified for further work included correlating the morphological changes that red blood cells undergo during hemolysis that were observed *in vitro* with those observed *in vivo* and on the dermal uptake of BE vapor; each of which were eventually resolved with further research (need Udden's reference; Corley *et al.*, 1997). These discussions eventually set the stage for the organization of a collaborative EPA and industry steering team in 1995 to establish a new RfC and RfD for BE under EPA's program to revise the IRIS process.

A team of scientists from industry, consulting firms and EPA worked together from 1995 to 1997 to develop an IRIS support document for use by EPA. In addition to default procedures (procedures used prior to their draft 1990 revision as discussed above for the provisional RfC), the team developed RfC's and RfD's using a PBPK model, benchmark dose (BMD_{05})/benchmark concentration (BMC_{05}) calculations in lieu of animal NOELs, and a combined BMD/BMC-PBPK approach. These methods and supporting documents were evaluated and modified by EPA scientists following both an external and internal scientific peer review prior to finalization. The summary information and toxicology review in support of a RfC of 13 mg/m^3 and a RfD of 0.5 mg/kg/day for BE were finalized by EPA in 1999 and are accessible on the EPA IRIS web site (EPA, 1999). The basis for these calculations are summarized below.

Oral Reference Dose (RfD) calculations. Since no chronic oral studies were available for BE, the principle study supporting the development of an oral RfD was the NTP subchronic drinking water study (NTP, 1993). In this study, groups of 10 male and female rats and mice were exposed to BE via their drinking water at concentrations of 0, 750, 1500, 3000, 4500 or 6000 ppm for 13 weeks. Rats were more sensitive than mice with effects primarily associated with hemolysis observed. A NOAEL for hematological effects was not identified in rats. Therefore, the lowest dose, 750 ppm in water or 54.9 and 58.6 mg/kg/day, was considered a LOAEL for hemolysis in male and female rats, respectively. Changes in the mean corpuscular volume (MCV; an indicator of erythrocyte swelling and increased numbers of reticulocytes) and red blood cell count (RBC; an indicator of cell lysis) were used as earliest measurable hemolytic responses (critical effects) for both oral and inhalation exposures to BE.

Once the principle study (NTP, 1993) and critical effects (MCV and RBC) were defined, RfD's were calculated by determining human equivalent doses (HED) then applying uncertainty factors (UF) to account for uncertainties associated with extrapolation from experimental conditions to the assumed human exposure scenario (e.g. chronic exposure over a lifetime). Uncertainty factors consisted of human to sensitive human (UF_H), animal to human (UF_A), subchronic to chronic (UF_S), LOAEL to NOAEL (UF_L) and incomplete database (UF_D) with a final modifying factor (MF) for the overall quality of the database.

Human equivalent doses were calculated using four methods: standard default, BMD, PBPK, and combined PBPK/BMD. For standard default calculations, no adjustments were made to the animal LOAEL for the HED since drinking water exposures were continuous in the NTP (1993) critical study. The male LOAEL (54.9 mg/kg/day) was chosen for this calculation as it was the more conservative of the two LOAEL's.

Benchmark dose analyses of the two critical effects (MCV and RBC) from the NTP study resulted in a steeper dose-response curve for MCV; thus dose-response information on MCV was used to derive the RfD. Although the male rats had a slightly lower LOAEL than females, the BMD analysis indicated a steeper dose-response curve for females. Thus, data from females were used in all BMD- and PBPK-based oral RfD's. For deriving the RfD, the MCV data were evaluated as continuous data; thus BMD_{05} was considered a more appropriate basis than BMD_{10}. Using the 95% lower confidence limit of the dose-response curve from the power model, the BMD_{05} was determined to be 49 mg/kg/day. As with the standard default procedure, this value was also considered to be the HED because animals were continuously exposed to BE via their drinking water.

For the PBPK-based HED, the Corley *et al.* (1994) PBPK model was used to derive the HED for the oral RfD using peak blood concentrations

(Cmax) for BAA as the internal dose metric. Three steps were involved in calculating the HED corresponding to the animal LOAEL: (1) calculate BAA blood Cmax corresponding to the female rat LOAEL assuming drinking water was consumed only during a 12-hr awake cycle on a 7 day/week schedule in simulations; (2) verify that steady-state was achieved (e.g. no change in Cmax as a result of prolonging the exposure regimen); (3) determine the amount of BE consumed by a human (HED, mg/kg/day) that resulted in the same Cmax for BAA in blood determined in step 1, assuming a 70 kg human consumes an average of 2 L/day during a 12-hr awake cycle. The Cmax for BAA in blood of female rats exposed to 58.6 mg/kg/day over 13 weeks determined by the PBPK model was 103 μM. The human equivalent dose corresponding to this Cmax ($LOAEL_{HED}$) was 7.6 mg/kg/day.

For the combined BMD/PBPK approach, the Cmax for BAA in blood, determined by the Corley *et al.* (1994) model, were used in place of administered doses in the BMD analysis of MCV data. The resulting BMD_{05} at the 95% lower confidence limit was 64 μM BAA. The PBPK model was then used to calculate the amount of BE consumed by humans in their drinking water during a 12-hr awake cycle on a daily basis that corresponded to this Cmax, or 5.1 mg/kg/day.

A default value of 10 was selected to account for variation in sensitivity within the human population (UF_H) for all of the RfD calculations. Although several *in vitro* studies and poisoning case reports have indicated that the elderly and patients with fragile red blood cells would not be more sensitive to the hemolytic effects of BE than normal adults and laboratory animals (see Udden, 1995 for summary), EPA considered information on potential hemolytic effects in humans over a broad range of exposure conditions or with individuals predisposed to hemolytic anemia or infants to be inadequate to warrant reduction of the UF_H below the default value. However, recent preliminary results from an ongoing CMA-sponsored research program investigating potentially sensitive human subgroups indicates that young children may not be any more sensitive to BAA-induced hemolysis than adults. In this study no hemolysis was observed in blood samples collected from 20 children, ranging in ages ranging from newborn to 35 months, at concentrations of BAA as high as 10 mM, which cannot be achieved following environmental exposures (Dr. Mark Udden, personal communication). Additional work is in progress to expand this database.

The uncertainty factor for interspecies (animal to human) variation (UF_A) accounts for pharmacodynamic and pharmacokinetic differences between animals and humans and thus, partial uncertainty factors (e.g. $10^{1/2}$ or ~3) have recently been utilized. Several *in vivo* and *in vitro* studies indicate that humans are less sensitive than rats (Carpenter *et al.* 1956; Ghanayem and Sullivan, 1993; Udden and Patton, 1994; Udden, 1994), thus a fractional component (e.g. <1) for the pharmacodynamic component of the UF_A was considered. However, the *in vivo* relative sensitivity could not be quantitiated. Thus, a value of 1 was used to account for pharmacodynamic differences between rats and humans for all RfD calculations. For the standard default and BMD approaches, an overall UF_A of 3 (1 for pharmacodynamics and 3 for pharmacokinetics) was used. For the PBPK and combined BMD/PBPK approaches, an overall UF_A of 1 was used since the pharmacokinetic differences were already accounted for by the use of the PBPK model.

For all RfD calculation approaches, a value of 1 was used for extrapolating the results from a subchronic study to chronic exposures (UF_S). Although no chronic oral studies were available, rats appear to develop tolerance to BE-induced hemolysis (Ghanayem *et al.*, 1992) and there was not a significant increase in the severity of hemolysis beyond 1-3 weeks of oral (NTP, 1993) or inhalation (NTP, 1998) exposures.

For the standard default and PBPK approaches, a value of 3 was selected for extrapolating a LOAEL to a NOAEL (UF_L). A value less than the default of 10 was used since the LOAEL was very near the threshold for the hemolytic effects of concern. For BMD and combined BMD/PBPK approaches a value of 1 was used for the UF_L because of the minimal and precursive nature of the critical effect (cell swelling as measured by increased MCV) and the fact that a BMD_{05} for a minimally adverse effect is generally treated like a NOAEL for continuous data sets.

A value of 1 was used for the database UF_D for all methods of analysis. While no chronic oral studies or adequate human data were available for BE, oral and inhalation (including chronic exposures) dose-response data indicated that there would be little, if any, increase in severity of hemolytic effects beyond subchronic exposure durations. In addition, there were chronic and subchronic studies available in two species (rats and mice) and adequate reproductive and developmental studies as well as limited studies in humans following short-term inhalation exposures. A modifying factor of 1 was used for all approaches.

The final RfD of 0.5 mg/kg/day was based upon the combined BMD/PBPK method since this approach incorporated much of the mechanistic information available for BE, best characterized the dose-response relationships between BE and hemolysis and reduced the uncertainties to the greatest extent. A summary of the four approaches is provided in Table 2.

Inhalation Reference Concentration (RfC) calculations. The principal studies supporting the inhalation RfC were the NTP subchronic and chronic inhalation studies in rats and mice (NTP, 1998). In the subchronic portion of NTP's chronic inhalation bioassay, both F344/N rats and B6C3F1 mice were exposed to 0, 31, 62.5, 125, 250 or 500 ppm BE for 6 hr/day, 5 days/week for 14 weeks; in the chronic study, rats were exposed to 0, 31, 62.5 or 125

Table 2. Summary of four methods for determination of an oral RfD for BE.

	Approach			
Parameter	**Standard**	**BMD_{05}**	**PBPK**	**BMD_{05}/PBPK**
Animal LOAEL (mg/kg/day)	55 (male rat)	NA (female rat)	59	NA
HED (mg/kg/day)	55	58	7.6	5.1
UF_H	10	10	10	10
UF_A	3	3	1	1
UF_S	1	1	1	1
UF_L	3	1	3	1
UF_D	1	1	1	1
MF	1	1	1	1
$UF_{(Total)}$	100	30	30	10
RfD (mg/kg/day)	**0.6**	**2**	**0.3**	**0.5**

ppm BE while mice were exposed to 0, 62.5, 125 or 250 ppm BE for 6 hr/day, 5 days/week for 2 years (NTP, 1998). Hematological parameters were evaluated in various groups of rats and mice after 3, 6 and 12 months of exposure. The critical effect for RfC calculations (MCV and RBC) were the same as those used in the oral RfD. Female rats were considered the most sensitive with a LOAEL of 31 ppm; a NOAEL was not identified. As with the oral RfD, human equivalent concentrations (HEC) and RfC's were calculated using four different methods.

There were two steps involved in the standard default approach to calculating a HEC from the female rat LOAEL. First, the units from the LOAEL in the animal exposure (31 ppm) were converted to 150 mg/m^3. This LOAEL is then multiplied by the ratio of the rat and human blood:air partition coefficients for BE. In this case, the default ratio of 1 was used. This value, 150 mg/m^3, was considered the HEC and was not adjusted for less than continuous exposures (e.g. multiplied by 6 hr/24 hr x 5 days/7 days) as was done in the 1991 provisional RfC since dose-rate was considered more important to BE toxicity than total dose.

For the BMC approach, both the MCV and RBC count response data were evaluated in female rats for all exposure durations studied by NTP in their subchronic and chronic bioassays and the Dodd *et al.* (1983) subchronic study. Similar to the oral RfD, the BMC_{05} was considered more appropriate than the BMC_{10}, since these endpoints were evaluated as continuous data. The steepest concentration-response curves (and lowest BMC_{05}

estimates) were obtained for decreased RBC counts in female rats. Since the severity of the effect did not change with increasing exposure duration (3, 6 and 12 months), the best fit model (BMDS polynomial model) obtained for the NTP 14-week subchronic female rat exposures (excluding the two highest exposure concentrations, 250 and 500 ppm) was used as the basis for the HEC. The BMC_{05} determined from these data was 27 ppm (130 mg/m^3) using the 95% lower confidence limit. This estimated BMC_{05} was considered the HEC and was not adjusted for less than continuous exposures as with the standard default approach.

For the PBPK-based approach, the Lee *et al.* (1998) PBPK model was used to derive the internal dose metric, Cmax for BAA (285 μM) corresponding to the female rat LOAEL (31 ppm) using the same procedures described for the RfD. The Lee *et al.* model was used for this calculation since it was formulated specifically to describe the kinetics of BE and BAA under the exposure conditions used in the NTP study. The HEC for continuous human exposures that resulted in this same Cmax at steady-state was calculated with the PBPK model of Corley *et al.* (1997). This HEC (98 ppm) was then converted to units of 474 mg/m^3 for RfC calculations.

For the combined BMC/PBPK approach, the Cmax for BAA in blood in female rats determined by the Lee *et al.* (1998) model, were used in place of actual exposure concentrations in the BMC analysis of RBC count data. The resulting BMC_{05} at the 95% lower confidence limit was 225 μM BAA. The Corley *et al.* (1997) model was then used to calculate a continuous human exposure that resulted in this same Cmax at steady-state. (HEC = 78 ppm or 380 mg/m3) for RfC calculations.

As with the oral RfD, a value of 10 was used to account for the variation in sensitivity within the human population (UF_H); a value of 1 was used for for extrapolating the results from subchronic to chronic exposures (UF_S); a value of 1 was used for the database (UF_D); and a partial uncertainty factor of 1 was used to account for the pharmacodynamic differences between rats and humans (UF_A) in all RfC calculations. An overall UF_A of 1 was used to account for both pharmacokinetic and pharmacodynamic differences in all RfC calculations since each approach for an inhalation RfC accounted for pharmacokinetic differences by either PBPK or default methods. For all calculations, a value of 3 was selected for extrapolating a LOAEL or BMC estimate to a NOAEL (UF_L). A modifying factor of 1 was also used in all approaches.

The use of a UF_L of 3 appears to be a relatively recent modification to the philosophy of using benchmark concentration calculations which, in the past, had generally been treated as equivalent to the NOAEL. However, a UF_L of 3 in the RfC was negotiated in response to a concern during EPA's consensus review that reduced RBC counts was considered a more severe effect

Table 3. Summary of four methods for determination of an inhalation RfC for BE.

	Approach			
Parameter	**Standard**	**BMC_{05}**	**PBPK**	**BMC_{05}/PBPK**
Animal LOAEL (mg/m^3) (female rat)	150 (female rat)	NA	150	NA
HEC (mg/m^3)	150	130	474	380
UF_H	10	10	10	10
UF_A	1	1	1	1
UF_S	1	1	1	1
UF_L	3	3	3	3
UF_D	1	1	1	1
MF	1	1	1	1
$UF_{(Total)}$	30	30	30	30
RfC (mg/m^3)	**5**	**4**	**16**	**13**

than increased MCV (the basis for the oral RfD) and that a 5% change in a toxic endpoint may not be acceptable. This procedural shift is likely to stimulate debate both inside and outside the EPA.

The final RfC of 13 mg/m^3 was based upon the combined BMD/PBPK method since this approach incorporated much of the mechanistic information available for BE, best characterized the dose-response relationships between BE and hemolysis and reduced the uncertainties to the greatest extent. A summary of the four approaches is provided in Table 3.

2.6 Conclusions

PBPK modeling has enabled the integration of numerous studies on the kinetics of BE in rats, mice and humans following a variety of exposure scenarios with an extensive mode of action and toxicity database. As a result, the scientific basis for human health risk assessments and the confidence in exposure guidelines for BE have been significantly improved. PBPK models were used to not only determine the concentrations to which humans must be exposed to result in the same internal doses associated with no-effect and effect levels in animal studies but also to modify uncertainty factors used in establishing exposure levels without an appreciable risk. As additional mechanism or modes of action studies are completed, internal dose metrics (Cmax and AUC for BAA in blood) may be further refined to improve the accuracy and continue the reduction in the uncertainty associated with the extrapolation of results from animals studies to realistic human exposures.

2.7 Acknowledgments

In addition to the authors, the following members of the Chemical Manufacturers Association (CMA)/EPA steering team made significant contributions to the toxicological review and methods for determination of the RfC and RfD for BE: Drs. Vicki Dellarco (EPA), Rodney Boatman (Kodak) and Dennis Paustenbach (Exponent). The CMA Ethylene Glycol Ethers Panel is also acknowledged for their support in the development of the PBPK model and other mechanistic research with BE. Numerous people provided advice and support for the development of the PBPK model including Dan Markham and Gary Bormett of Dow Chemical, Drs. Jean-Marie Houle and Amanda Masterman (LAB/BioResearch), Dr. Burhan Ghanayem (NIEHS), Dr. Gunnar Johanson (NIOH, Sweden), Drs. Pat Sabourin, Karla Thrall, Monica Lee of Battelle and Dr. Donna Grant (Purdu Pharma) and are gratefully acknowledged.

2.8 References

Agency for Toxic Substances and Disease Registry (ATSDR). (1999). Toxicological profile for 2-butoxyethanol and 2-butoxyethanol acetate. Division of Toxicology, Toxicology Information Branch, Publication PB/99/102527/AS. Atlanta, GA.

Andersen, M. E., Clewell III, H. J., Gargas, M. L., Smith, F. A., and Reitz, R. H. (1987). Physiologically-based pharmacokinetics and the risk assessment process for methylene chloride. *Toxicol. Appl. Pharmacol.* 87, 185-205.

Bachowski, S., Xu, Y., Stevenson, D.E., Walbork, E.F. Jr. and Klaunig, J.E. (1998). Role of oxidative stress in the selective toxicity of dieldrin in the mouse liver. *Toxicol. Appl. Pharmacol.* 150, 301-309.

Bormett, G., Bartels, M.J. and Markham, D.A. (1995). Determination of 2-Butoxyethanol and butoxyacetic acid in rat and human blood by gas chromatography/mass spectrometry. *J. Chromatog. B.* 665, 315-325.

Carpenter, C.P., Pozzani, U.C., Weil, C.S., Nair III, J.H., Keck, G.A. and Smyth Jr., H.F. (1956). The toxicity of butyl cellosolve solvent. *A.M.A. Arch. Ind. Health.* 14, 114-131.

CEFIC. (1995). Document 486/95/7/STAT/YEAR, *Oxygenated Solvents S.G.-Statistical Investigation: 1994,* dated February 23, 1995.

Chemical Manufacturers Association (CMA) (1997). *BE A World of Solutions.* A review of the uses and health effects of ethylene glycol nomobutyl ether. CMA. Washington, D.C.

Corley, R. A., Bormett, G. A. and Ghanayem, B.I. 1994. Physiologically-based pharmacokinetics of 2-butoxyethanol and its major metabolite, 2-butoxyacetic acid, in rats and humans. *Toxicol. Appl. Pharmacol.* 129, 61-79.

Corley, R.A., Markham, D.A., Banks, C., Delorme, P., Masterman, A. and Houle, J.M. (1997). Physiologically-based pharmacokinetics and the dermal absorption of 2-butoxyethanol vapor by humans. *Fund. Appl. Toxicol.* 39, 120-130.

Dill, J.A., Lee, M.K., Bates, D.J., Anderson, D.J., Johnson, R.E., Chou, B.J., Burka, L.T. and Roycroft, J.H. (1998). Toxicokinetics of inhaled 2-butoxyethanol and its major metabolite, 2-butoxyacetic acid, in F344 rats and B6C3F1 mice. *Toxicol. Appl. Pharmacol.* 153, 227-242.

Dodd, D.E., Snellings, W.M., Maronpot, R.R. and Ballantyne, B. (1983). Ethylene glycol monobutyl ether: acute, 9-day and 90-day vapor inhalation studies in Fischer 344 rats. *Toxicol. Appl. Pharmacol.* 68, 405-414.

ECETOC. (1994). European Chemical Industry Ecology and Toxicology Centre. Special Report No. 7. Butoxyethanol Criteria Document Including a Suplement for 2-Butoxyethyl Acetate. April, 1994. Brussels, Belgium.

Environmental Protection Agency (EPA). (1994). Methods for derivation of inhalation reference concentrations and application of inhalation dosimetry. United States Environmental Protection Agency, Office of Health and Environmental Assessment, Washington, D.C. October, 1994. EPA/600/8-90/066F.

Environmental Protection Agency (EPA). (1999). Toxicological Review of Ethylene Glycol Monobutyl Ether (EGBE). United States Environmental Protection Agency, In Support of Summary Information on the Integrated Risk Information System (IRIS; http://www.epa.gov/iris). October, 1999.

Farris, E.J. (1998). Age-, Gender- and Species-Comparison of Blood and Tissue Partition Coefficients for 2-Butoxyacetic Acid. Masters Thesis. Washington State University.

Ghanayem, B.I. (1989). Metabolic and cellular basis of 2-butoxyethanol-induced hemolytic anemia in rats and assessment of human risk in vitro. Biochem. Pharmacol. 38, 1679-1684.

Ghanayem, B.I., Burka, L.T. and Matthews, H.B. (1987a). Metabolic basis of ethylene glycol monobutyl ether (2-butoxyethanol) toxicity: role of alcohol and aldehyde dehydrogenases. J. Pharmacol. Exp. Therap. 242, 222-231.

Ghanayem, B.I., Burka, L.T., Sanders, J.M. and Matthews, H.B. (1987b). Metabolism and disposition of ethylene glycol monobutyl ether (2-butoxyethanol) in rats. Drug Metab. Disp. 15, 478-484.

Ghanayem, B.I., Sanchez, I.M. and Matthews, H.B. (1992). Development of tolerance to 2-butoxyethanol-induced hemolytic anemia and studies to elucidate the underlying mechanisms. Toxicol. Appl. Pharmacol. 112, 198-206.

Ghanayem, B.I., Sanders, J.M., Clark, A.M., Bailer, J. and Matthews, H.B. (1990). Effects of dose, age, inhibition of metabolism and elimination on the toxicokinetics of 2-butoxyethanol and its metabolites. J. Pharmacol. Exp. Therap. 253, 136-143.

Ghanayem, B.I. and Sullivan, C.A. (1993). Assessment of the haemolytic activity of 2-butoxyethanol and its major metabolite, butoxyacetic acid, in various mammals including humans. Human and Exp. Toxicol. 12, 305-311.

Grant, D.M., Corley, R.A. and Thrall, K.D. (1997). A Comparison of Gender, Age, and Species Differences in Renal Active Secretion of 2-Butoxyacetic Acid. 8th An. North Amer. ISSX Meeting. Hilton Head, SC. Oct. 26-30, 1997.

Grant, D.M., Weitz, K.K., Corley, R.A. and Thrall, K.D. (1998). Gender-, Age- and Species-Dependent Differences in Metabolism of 2-Butoxyethanol Using Precision Cut Liver Slices. Abst. #1624. 37th An. Society of Toxicology Meeting. Seattle, WA. March 1-5, 1998.

Gualtieri, J.F., Harris, C.R, Corley, R.A., Markham, D.A., Roy, R.R, and Manderfield, C.E. (1995). Multiple 2-butoxyethanol intoxications in the same patient: clinical findings, pharmacokinetics, and therapy. North American Congress of Clinical Toxicology. Rochester, NY.

Johanson, G. (1986). Physiologically based pharmacokinetic modeling of inhaled 2-butoxyethanol in man. Toxicol. Lett. 34, 23-31.

Johanson, G. (1989). Analysis of ethylene glycol ether metabolites in urine by extractive alkylation and electron-capture gas chromatography. Arch. Toxicol. 63, 107-111.

Johanson, G. (1994). Inhalation toxicokinetics of butoxyethanol and its metabolite butoxyacetic acid in the male Sprague-Dawley rat. Toxicology. 68, 588-594.

Johanson, G. and Boman, A. (1991). Percutaneous absorption of 2-butoxyethanol vapour in human subjects. Br. J. Indust. Med. 48, 788-792.

Johanson, G. and Dynesius, B. (1988). Liquid/air partition coefficients of six commonly used glycol ethers. Br. J. Indust. Med. 45, 561-564.

Johanson, G. and Johnsson, S. (1991). Gas chromatographic determination of butoxyacetic acid in human blood after exposure to 2-butoxyethanol. Arch. Toxicol. 65, 433-435.

Johanson, G., Boman, A., and Dynesius, B. (1988). Percutaneous absorption of 2-butoxyethanol in man. Scand. J. Work Environ. Health. 14, 101-109.

Johanson, G., Kronborg, H., Naslund, P.H., Nordqvist, M.B. (1986a). Toxicokinetics of inhaled 2-butoxyethanol (ethylene glycol monobutyl ether) in man. Scand. J. Environ. Hlth. 12, 594-602.

Johanson, G., Wallen, M., and Nordquist, M. B. (1986b). Elimination kinetics of 2-butoxyethanol in the perfused rat liver--dose dependence and effect of ethanol. Toxicol. Appl. Pharmacol. 83, 315-320.

Lee, M.K., Dill, J.A., Chou, B.J. and Roycroft, J.H. (1998). Physiologically based pharmacokinetic model for chronic inhalation of 2-butoxyethanol. Toxicol. Appl. Pharmacol. 153, 211-226.

Lee, M.K., Stenner, R.D., Corley, R.A. and Thrall, K.D. (1995). A physiologically based pharmacokinetic (PBPK) model for 2-butoxyethanol and its hemolytic metabolite, 2-butoxyacetic acid. Abstract 63-PF-2. VII International Congress of Toxicology. July 2-6, 1995. Seattle, WA.

Markham, D.A., Bartels, M.J., Corley, R.A. and Rettenmeier, A.W. (1995). Analysis of 2-butoxyethanol and metabolites in human urine by GC & ESI/MS. Abst. #WPG 170. 43rd ASMS Conference on Mass Spectrometry and Allied Topics. May 21-26, 1995.

Medinsky, M.A., Singh, G., Bechtold, W.E., Bond, J.A., Sabourin, P.J., Birnbaum, L.S., and Henderson, R.F. (1990). Disposition of three glycol ethers in drinking water to male F344/N rats. Toxicol. Appl. Pharmacol. 102, 443-455.

Mordenti, J. (1986). Man versus beast: Pharmacokinetic scaling in mammals. J. Pharm. Sci. 75, 1028-1040.

National Institute for Occupational Safety and Health (NIOSH). (1990). Occupational exposure to ethylene glycol monobutyl ether and ethylene glycol monobutyl ether acetate. Criteria for a recommended standard. DHHS (NIOSH) Publication No. 90-118.

National Toxicology Program (NTP). (1998). Technical report on the toxicology and carcinogenesis studies of 2-butoxyethanol (CAS No. 111-76-2) in F344/N rats and B6C3F1 mice (inhalation studies). U.S. Department of Health and Human Services, Public Health Service, National Institutes of Health, Research Triangle Park, NC. NTP TR 484. NIH Draft Publication No. 98-3974.

National Toxicology Program (NTP). (1993). Technical report on toxicity studies of ethylene glycol ethers 2-methoxyethanol, 2-ethoxyethanol, 2-butoxyethanol administered in drinking water to F344/N rats and B6C3F1 mice. U.S. Department of Health and Human Services, Public Health Service, National Institutes of Health, Research Triangle Park, NC. NTP No. 26. NIH Publication No. 93-3349.

Rettenmeier, A.W., Hennigs, R. and Wodarz, R. (1993). Determination of butoxyacetic acid and N-butoxyacetylglutamine in urine of lacquerers exposed to 2-butoxyethanol. Int. Arch. Occup. Environ. Health 65, S151-S153.

Sabourin, P.J., Medinsky, M.A., Birnbaum, L.S., Griffith, W.C. and Henderson, R.F. (1992a). Effect of exposure concentration on the disposition of inhaled butoxyethanol by F344 rats. Toxicol. Appl. Pharmacol. 114, 232-238.

Sabourin, P.J., Medinsky, M.A., Thurmond, F., Birnbaum, L.S. and Henderson, R.F. (1992b). Effect of dose on the disposition of methoxyethanol, ethoxyethanol, and butoxyethanol administered dermally to male F344/N rats. Fund. Appl. Toxicol. 19, 124-132.

Shyr, L.J., Sabourin, P.J., Medinsky, M.A., Birnbaum, L.S. and Henderson, R.F. (1993). Physiologically-based modeling of 2-butoxyethanol disposition in rats following different routes of exposure. Env. Res. 63, 202-218.

Sivarao, D.V. and Mehendele, H.M. (1995). 2-Butoxyethanol autoprotection is due to resiliance of newly formed erythrocytes to hemolysis. Arch. Toxicol. 69, 526-532.

Tyler, T.R. (1984). Acute and subchronic toxicity of ethylene glycol monobutyl ether. Environ. Health Persp. 57, 185-191.

Udden, M. M. (1994). Hemolysis and decreased deformability of erythrocytes exposed to butoxyacetic acid, a metabolite of 2-butoxyethanol: II. Resistance in red blood cells from humans with potential susceptibility. J. Appl. Toxicol. 14, 97-102.

Udden, MM. (1995) Effects of butoxyacetic acid on human red cells. Occup. Hyg. 2, 283-292.

Udden, M. M. and Patton, C. S. (1994). Hemolysis and decreased deformability of erythrocytes exposed to butoxyacetic acid, a metabolite of 2-butoxyethanol. I. Sensitivity in rats and resistance in normal humans. J. Appl. Toxicol. 14, 91-96.

Werner H.W., Mitchell, J.L., Miller, J.W. and von Oettingen, W.F. (1943a). Effects of repeated exposure of dogs to monoalkyl ethylene glycol ether vapors. J. Ind. Hyg. Toxicol. 25, 409.

Werner, H.W., Mitchell, J.L., Miller, J.W. and von Oettingen, W.F. (1943b). The acute toxicity of vapors of several monoalkyl ethers of ethylene glycol. J. Ind. Hyg. Toxicol. 25, 157-163.

Werner, H.W., Nawrocki, C.Z., Mitchell, J.L., Miller, J.W. and von Oettingen, W.F. (1943c). Effects of repeated exposure of rats to vapors of monoalkyl ethylene glycol ethers. J. Ind. Hyg. Toxicol. 25, 374-379.

Worksafe Australia. (1996). National Industrial Chemicals Notification and Assessment Scheme (NICNAS) Summary Report: 2-Butoxyethanol in cleaning products. Australian Government Publishing Service, GPO Box 84, Canberra ACT 2601.

World Health Organization (WHO). (1998). Concise International Chemical Assessment Document (CICAD) No. 10. 2-Butoxyethanol. Geneva, Switzerland.

Xue, H., Kamendulis, L.M. and Klaunig, J.E. (1999). A potential mechanism for 2-butoxyethanol (2-BE) induced mouse liver neoplasia. Toxicol. Sci. 1-S, 231.

3 APPLICATION OF PHARMACOKINETIC MODELLING TO BIOLOGICAL MONITORING

PIERRE O.DROZ

Scientist, Inst. for Occupational Health Sciences, Lausanne Univ., Switzerland

3.1 Introduction

Exposure monitoring is one of the key steps in the assessment of occupational risks. It is further very often used in risk management to monitor the performance of the controls in workplaces. Exposure can occur in workplaces via several different routes : inhalation, ingestion, dermal contact. However it is often perceived as airborne exposure, and is in most cases estimated via air monitoring. Air monitoring has several limitations in the estimation of total exposure:

(1) as mentioned, other routes of exposure exist, depending on the chemicals and to the exposure situation ;
(2) workers often use personal protective equipment and the efficiency of this equipment cannot be estimated by air monitoring;
(3) physical activity is known to increase pulmonary ventilation and thus uptake of chemicals, which is not reflected in air monitoring results;
(4) occupational exposures fluctuate widely over time, for example from one day to the next, and this requires repeated air sampling to estimate the average long term exposure:
(5) individual differences are known to exist between workers, for instance in body build or ability to metabolise chemicals, and these will have an impact on the level of active species at the site of action.

Biological monitoring of exposure can, at least partly, overcome these limitations. It consists of taking measurements of chemicals or their metabolites in body fluids, and therefore it takes into account other routes of exposure, the protection afforded by personal protection, the influence of physical exercise on uptake, individual differences in the handling of chemicals, and in some situations it reduces the uncertainties produced by the day-to-day exposure variability.

Occupational exposure is not continuous and usually follows an 8/16 hour cycle with periodic interruptions due to the weekend breaks. On the other hand, uptake and distribution of chemicals in the body is a kinetic

J. Krüse, H.J.M. Verhaar, and W.K. de Raat (eds.), The Practical Applicability of Toxicokinetic Models in the Risk Assessment of Chemicals, 41-53.

process which can, in a first approximation, be considered exponential. Furthermore, the use of biological monitoring to assess occupational exposure is complicated by the variability in biological levels of chemicals which can be observed both as a function of time, and at a given time between individuals. The combination of these aspects explains the importance of toxicokinetics in the development of biological monitoring techniques.

The objective of this chapter is to present some of the contributions of toxicokinetic modelling in the context of biological monitoring. Although toxicokinetics is of course inherent to every study on biological monitoring, the discussion will be restricted here to the use of pharmacokinetic models, and to their contribution to the understanding of the basis of biological monitoring of occupational exposure.

3.2 Biological Monitoring

Biological monitoring can be defined as the assessment of total exposure to a chemical or a defined mixture through measurements of an indicator in a body fluid. In case of occupational exposure, urine, blood and expired air are mainly used for biological-monitoring purposes. The indicator can be either the chemical itself (solvents in blood, metals in urine) or a metabolite (solvent metabolite in urine), or a characteristic reversible biochemical change induced by the chemical (sister chromatid exchanges, mutagenic activity in urine, thioether urinary excretion). Biological monitoring has to be distinguished here from health or medical surveillance which is aimed at detecting and measuring health effects. In the definition used here, it is a monitoring tool for exposure assessment.

The routine application of biological monitoring requires established reference values for interpretation. Such values are published in many countries by professional organisations or enforcement authorities. In the USA, the Biological Exposure Indices (BEI) committee of the American Conference of Governmental Industrial Hygienists (ACGIH) establishes reference values based on the concept that they are concentrations which are most likely found in workers exposed at the Threshold Limit Values (TLV-TWA) (ACGIH, 1999). BEIs are of course valid for a specified sampling time in relation to the exposure period. In Germany, the Deutsche Forschungsgemeinschaft publishes its own reference values, Biological Tolerance Values (BAT), which are considered the highest values which are equivalent to an exposure to the Maximum Workplace Concentration (MAK) (DFG, 1999). Both BEIs and BAT values are established with the rationale shown in Figure 1.

Ideally, biological reference values should be developed considering the relationship between biological levels and health effects. However data are

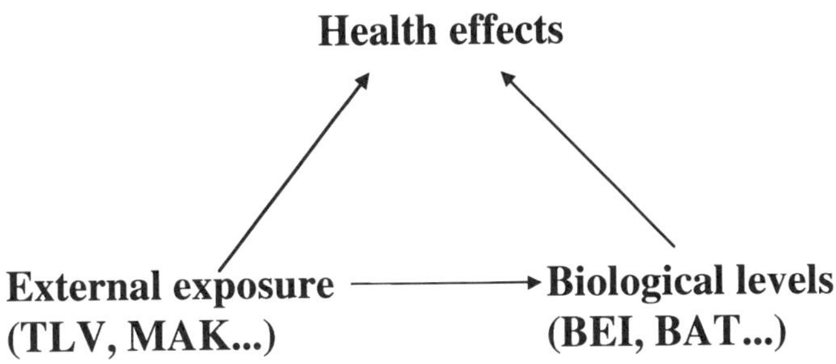

Figure 1. Functional relationships between external exposure, biological levels and health effects (for abbreviations see text).

often limited in this context and there is very much valuable information on the external exposure - health effect relationships. The external exposure - biological level link makes use of this fundamental information. Thus BEIs and BATs are often established as directly equivalent to a given external exposure (TLV or MAK).

In order to be able to develop sound biological monitoring programs, several aspects in relation with pharmacokinetics have to be considered. Sampling time is of course of utmost importance, and it depends largely on toxicokinetic considerations. But there are also other less evident aspects which should be considered and will be addressed here. The objective of this paper is to present a quick overview of some contributions of toxicokinetic modelling to biological monitoring.

Extrapolation to new situations. Often data exist from volunteer studies carried out at rest and for limited duration. The transition to occupational exposures can easily be done with modelling techniques.

Non-linear relationships with exposure. In most cases at the low exposures found in workplaces, toxicokinetics can be considered as linear. However, in some cases non-linear mechanisms come into play at these levels and should be analysed and taken into account.

3.3 Description of the Pharmacokinetic Models used

Pharmacokinetic models of different levels of sophistication can be used in the context of biological monitoring. The choice of the type of model, and of its detailed structure depends on the type of question which is addressed. For example when dealing with a specific chemical for which a large amount of information is available (affinities for the tissues, metabolic constants) a physiologically based pharmacokinetic (PBPK) model can be envisaged. On

Table 1. Physiological data, adjustment for body build, and physical workload (Droz *et al* 1989).

Compartment	Volume [% LBV]	Perfusion at rest [ml/min/ml]	Effect of physical workload [l/min]
Lungs			
tissue	0.9	Qb= Qi	Qi
air	5.5	Valv=0.8Qb	Valv+22 VO2
art. blood	1.9	-	-
Muscles and skin	69	33	Qi+7.4 VO2
Adipose tissues	FBV	22	Qi+ VO2
Brain	2.6	570	unchanged
Kidneys	0.53	4520	Qi(1-0.14 VO2)
Splanchnic	5.8	520	Qi(1-0.19 VO2)
Others	1.0	2830	unchanged
Venous blood	8.3	-	-

the other hand, when dealing with chemicals less studied, or when hoping to describe classes of compounds and trying to elaborate general rules, more simple models can be chosen in order to have less requirements for basic data.

For PBPK models, Table 1 summarises the main physiological input parameters required (Droz *et al,* 1989). To this list, one must add chemical specific parameters such as partition coefficients, Michaelis-Menten parameters and metabolites clearance data. In Table 1, physiological data for humans are expressed as a function of build and physical activity. This enables the simulation of different work situations, and of populations of workers with different characteristics.

For simpler toxicokinetic (TK) models, only some basic parameters are used such as: absorption rate, distribution volume, renal clearance or other routes of excretion. Several compartments can be used when required. They can either represent different chemicals (metabolites for example) or different tissues for a given chemical. Such simple models are well adapted to the description of the influence of various sources of variability on biological monitoring results. Table 2 summarises some data indicating the magnitude of variability for the main parameters of a TK model (Droz, 1992). Variability in absorption comes essentially from air exposure fluctuations (when uptake is by inhalation only) and from physical activity. For exposure, 3 situations are described with different coefficients of variation, as this depends on the situations and on the process (Droz, 1992).

Table 2. Examples of variability in a one-compartment model.

Parameters	Mean*	Coefficient of variation	Reference
Absorption			
low variability		0.18	Droz *et al* (1989)
medium variability		0.78	Droz *et al* (1989)
high variability		1.53	Droz *et al* (1989)
physical exercise (W)	43	0.46	Droz *et al* (1989)
Distribution			
body height (m)	1.77	0.041	NCHS (1981)
Quetelet index (kg/m2)	25.3	0.15	NCHS (1981)
peak		0.25	Hattis *et al* (1987)
Elimination			
half-life†		0.26	Hattis *et al* (1987)
AUC		0.34	Hattis *et al* (1987)

* When mean is not relevant, it is not indicated

† Half-life $T_{1/2}$ is a function of clearance Cl and distribution volume V_d

$$T_{1/2} = (V_d/\mathrm{Cl})\ln 2$$

3.4 Case Studies

3.4.1 Tetrahydrofuranet

Tetrahydrofurane (THF) is often used as a solvent in lacquers, glues, paints, inks and in the textile processing industry. Biological monitoring was suggested on several occasions for THF in the beginning of the 90s. In Germany, a biological tolerance value (BAT) of 8 mg/l was proposed for urine sampled at the end of the work shift (DFG, 1996). In the United States this substance was under study by the BEI Committee of ACGIH. However, divergences in the database available had precluded the establishment of a BEI. At least three studies on volunteers and one field study in workers were available for establishing a quantitative relationship between exposure and biological levels. Table 3 summarises these studies with the extrapolated biological levels for 200 ppm exposure. A large range of values is observed for all three biological media: breath, urine and blood. These differences could be due to different exposure protocols, and this possibility has been investigated with a PBPK model, with the hope to reconcile the differences.

Table 3. Extrapolated biological levels at 200 ppm from existing volunteer or field studies. Values have been estimated by linear extrapolation from available published information.

	Breath [ppm]	**Blood [mg/l]**	**Urine [mg/l]**	**Reference**
Workers	6.5	2.4	8	Ong *et al, 1991*
Volunteers at rest	2	-[a]	1.7	Teramoto *et al, 1994*
Volunteers with workload	21	10	8	Failing *et al, 1994*
Volunteers at rest	1.4	1.9	1.5	Cocker *et al, 1996*
Volunteers at rest	3.4	2.4	1.6	Teramoto *et al, 1994*

[a] data not usable because of unit uncertainties

A seven-compartment linear PBPK model was used (Table 1). Information on THF affinities for the tissue groups was obtained by *in vitro* measurement of partition coefficients. As no quantitative data were available concerning the metabolic rate of THF, it was assumed that metabolism was fast in the hepatic tissue, and therefore flow limited. Urinary excretion was simulated by glomerular filtration followed by passive reabsorption in the tubules according to the water (urine)-blood partition coefficient. Urinary excretion rate was calculated based on a daily creatinine excretion of 1.4 g.

To test the PBPK model, exposure scenarios used by several research groups were simulated. The results obtained are presented in Figure 2 for experimental exposures. It can be quickly seen that a fair agreement is obtained in two of the three studies available, both for urine and breath. In one case however the discrepancy is very large, and it is difficult to reconcile these results with the two other studies. A fair agreement is also reached when simulating repeated exposures of the workers (physical exercise 50W) and comparing the results to what was obtained in workers. The results predicted by the PBPK model and obtained in workers (in parentheses) at 200 ppm are 5.1 ppm (6.5 ppm), 56.9 mmol/l (33.0 mmol/l) and 100.3 mmol/l (111.9 mmol/l) for breath, blood and urine sampled at the end of work, respectively.

The PBPK model made it possible to reconcile three out of four studies carried out under different conditions (exposure: repeated versus single, subjects: volunteers versus workers, physical exercise: rest versus working conditions). It is not yet clear what happened to the third study, but the difference cannot be reduced to toxicokinetic factors. A simple PBPK model, based on a limited amount of data was therefore able to shed some light on apparently inconsistent results. Based on this, the simulation of 200 ppm repeated exposures including physical exercise produces a concentration in urine of 7.2 mg/l, very close to the BAT value of 8 mg/l.

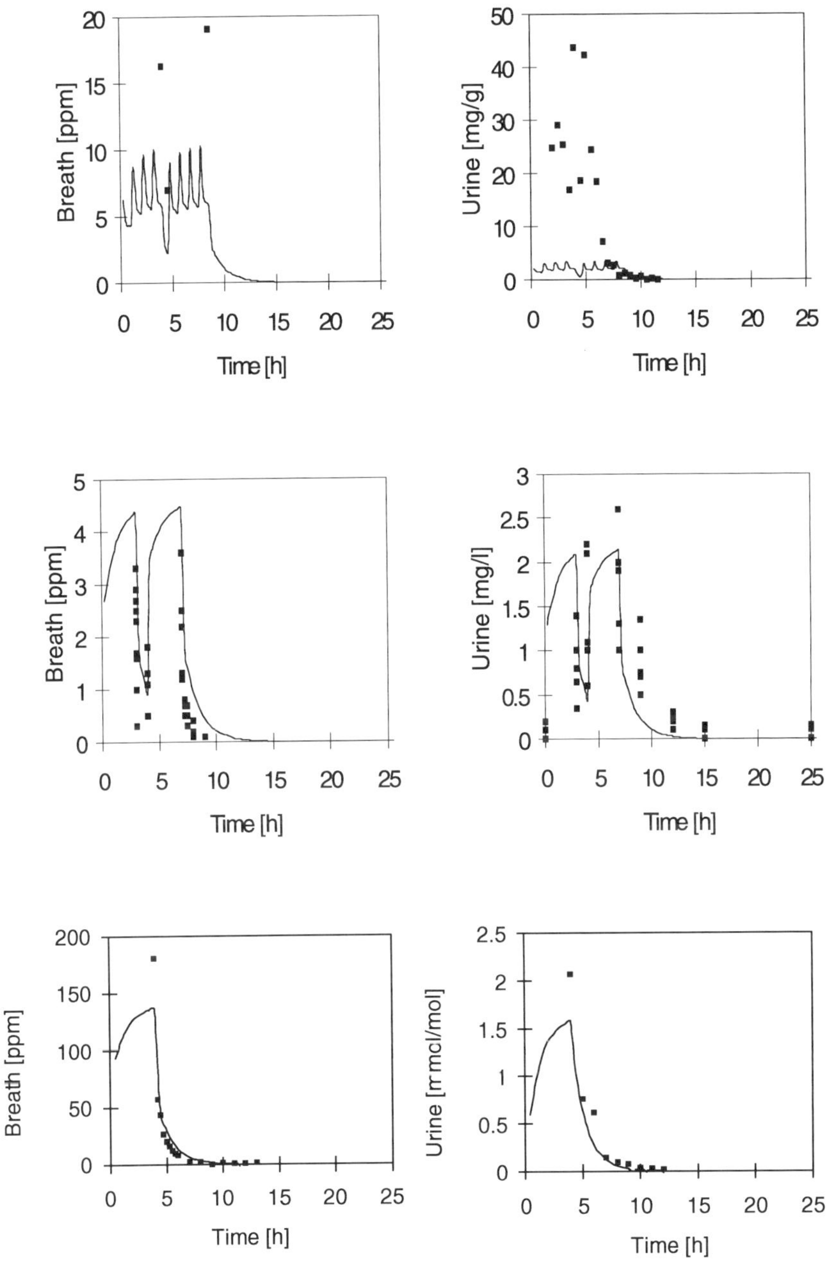

Figure 2. Comparison of model-predicted THF breath and urine concentrations with those measured in three independent experimental studies (top Cocker *et al* 1996, middle Teramoto *et al* 1997, bottom Failing *et al* 1994).

3.4.2 Formic Acid after Methyl Formate or Methanol Exposure

Methyl formate (MF) is used as a catalyst and binding agent for core sand in the production of mould cores in iron foundries. It is metabolised into methanol (MeOH) and formic acid (FA) by hydrolysis, either non-enzymatically or by esterases present in the plasma and other tissues. Besides ester cleavage, MF oxidation has also been shown, resulting in the production of formaldehyde (Fald) and FA. In the case of MeOH exposure or intake, there is considerable evidence that FA is the toxic species, and this probably applies also to MF. To protect against potential health effects, an exposure limit value of 100 ppm has been recommended by the ACGIH. Germany and other countries have recently adopted a 50 ppm limit.

Biological monitoring of MF exposure can be carried out by monitoring of urine for both MeOH and FA. Recent results have shown a tendency to nonlinear behaviour for FA (Figure 4). It was therefore decided to explore this possibility with a modelling approach to ascertain the biological moni-

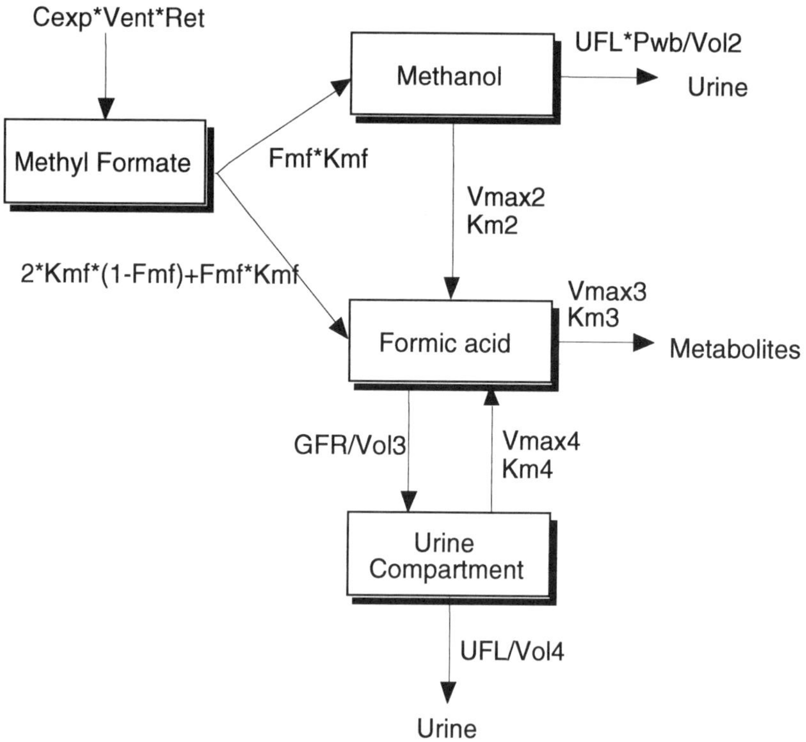

Figure 3. Schematic description of the TK model for MF (Nihlen et al 1999). Abbreviations : UFL, urine flow; Vol4, volume of urine compartment; GFR, glomerular filtration rate; Pwb, water-blood partition coefficient; Vol2, distribution volume of MeOH; Cexp, exposure concentration, Vent, ventilation rate; Ret, pulmonary retention; Fmf, fraction of MF; Kmf, rate constant of MF.

toring of MF better, and also to improve our understanding of MeOH monitoring. There has been a lot of discussion on the relevant use of FA as an indicator for exposure to MeOH (Franzblau *et al* 1997). From studies with workers FA seems to be a useful indicator but it does not show any increase after volunteer exposure.

The simple TK model shown in Figure 3 was build to describe the behaviour of MF in the body. To simplify the model, formaldehyde was not included as intermediate due to its short life in the body. FA could be produced either from MeOH or directly. Urinary excretion of MeOH was simulated by glomerular filtration and passive reabsorption as for THF above. For FA however, tubular reabsorption was included, but as a satur-able process, based on experimental data in animals (Damian 1996). All re-quired data for the TK model were available except for the proportion of MF undergoing oxidation rather than hydrolysis. This parameter was obtained by fitting to experimental data obtained during exposures in volunteers. It was shown that 85 to 97% of the metabolism occurred via hydrolysis.

The behaviour predicted by the TK model is shown in Figure 4 for MeOH and FA. Two scenarios are presented representing exposure at rest (0 W)

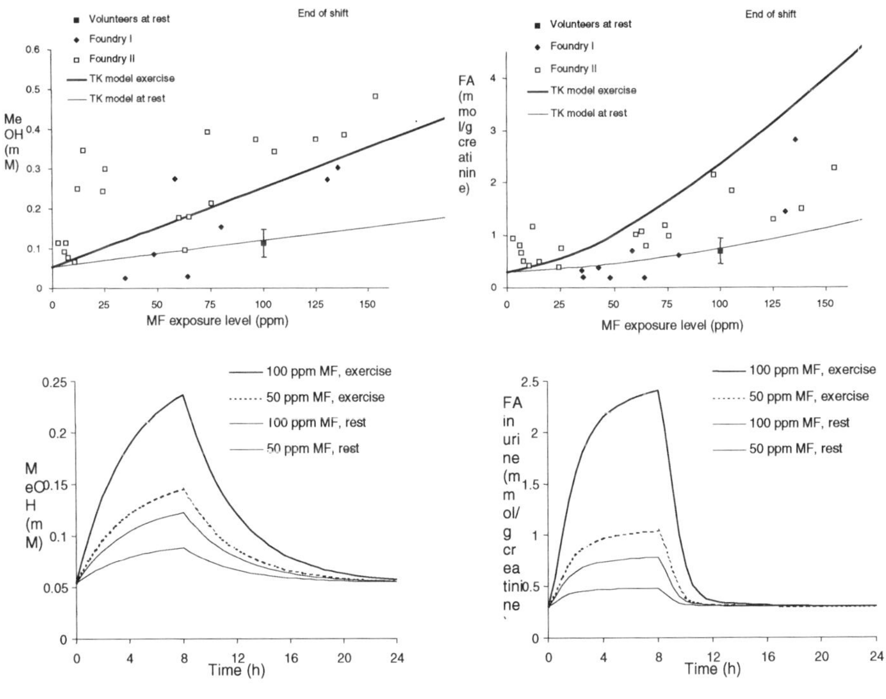

Figure 4. Predicted urinary excretions of MeOH and FA after occupational exposure to MF compared to actual measurements (top graphs) and after single experimental exposure under various conditions (Nihlen et al 1999).

and occupational exposure (50 W). Despite the large variability observed in the results, the TK model predicts biological levels well. It specifically demonstrates the non-linearity of FA as opposed to MeOH. This is further illustrated in Figure 4 (bottom) which shows the sudden increase in urinary FA above about 50 ppm exposure with physical exercise. This is due to the saturation of the reabsorption mechanism in the tubules.

With only slight modifications this TK model could be applied to MeOH exposure. As mentioned above data on urinary FA excretion from MeOH are divergent. On the one hand studies in workers have demonstrated an increase in urinary FA, on the other hand experimental exposures of volunteers have not been able to demonstrate this, except at high exposures (Table 4). One of the reasons could be the non-linear behaviour already simulated for FA from MF. The TK model was therefore applied here after deletion of the MF compartment and validation of its results with experimental data. In Table 4 for each study the predictions for both MeOH and FA are presented together with the literature data. For MeOH the agreement is rather satisfactory and increases are proportional to exposure. For FA in urine, it is generally seen that low exposures (in terms of concentration and physical workload) produce only marginal increases in the FA urinary excretions due to tubular reabsorption. On the other hand when exposure is elevated (physical exercise and inhaled concentrations), urinary FA excretion increases because of saturation in the mechanism of reabsorption. It eventually becomes high enough to be distinguished from background values. This general behaviour is seen qualitatively in both experimental and simulated results presented in Table 4. However a complete quantitative agreement is not reached in all cases and the TK model appears to overestimate the effect of high exposures. A complete agreement could possibly be reached by adjusting the non-linear constants which have been adopted from *in vitro* rat experiments.

3.5 Comments and Conclusion

It has been shown that models with variable degrees of complexity represent productive tools in the context of biological monitoring. They can be applied in many situations, either to understand the influence of selected variables such as physical workload, sampling time, metabolic capacity, or to act as predictor of biological levels in a given situation. Two successful examples of such applications have been given here in the fields of integration of various sources of experimental data collected under different protocols, and the understanding of the effect of non-linearity.

Toxicokinetic models can also be applied in other situations. For example the present tendency to move away from standard 8 hour work shifts has of course some impact on biological reference levels. The new levels can easily

Table 4. MeOH and FA excretion in urine after experimental and occupational exposure to MeOH. TK model predicted values and results from the literature (Nihlen *et al* 1999).

Methanol exposure	Number of objects	Exposure time	MeOH in urine after exposure mmol/l		FA in urine after exposure mmol/g creatinine		References
			Predicted	*Literature*	*Predicted*	*Literature*	
Volunteers							
0 ppm [b]	26	4 h	0.054	--	0.30	0.14 [c]	d'Alessandro, 1994
0 ppm [b]	11	8 h	0.054	0.047	0.30	0.26	Franzblau, 1997
0 ppm [d]	15	8 h	0.054	0.037	0.30	0.28	Franzblau, 1997
100 ppm [b]	12	8 h	0.20	0.27	0.39	0.37	Franzblau, 1997
100 ppm [d]	11	8 h	0.32	0.48	0.48	0.28	Franzblau, 1997
200ppm [b]	26	4 h	0.26	--	0.42	0.15 [c]	d'Alessandro, 1994
200 ppm [b]	1	4 h	0.26	0.20	0.42	0.31	Ogata, 1990
200 ppm [b]	11	8 h	0.34	0.56	0.50	0.33	Franzblau, 1997
200 ppm [d]	15	8 h	0.59	0.70	0.77	0.22	Franzblau, 1997
400 ppm [b]	11	8 h	0.64	0.95	0.83	0.61	Franzblau, 1997
400 ppm [d]	11	8 h	1.14	1.44	1.59	0.66	Franzblau, 1997
Workers							
85 ppm [a]	7	8 h	0.42	--	0.58	0.54 [c]	Angerer., 1997
93 ppm [a]	20	8 h	0.41	--	0.58	0.54 [c]	Heinrich. 1982
101 ppm [a]	8	8 h	0.49	--	0.66	0.46 [c]	Angerer, 1997
134 ppm [a]	6	8 h	0.64	--	0.84	0.34 [c]	Angerer, 1997

[a] workload of 50 W (worker).

[b] exposure at rest (volunteers).

[c] FA mmol/l, not corrected for creatinine.

[d] workload of 25 W (volunteers).

be estimated on the base of toxicokinetic considerations with models. Another example is the understanding of the interactions in exposures to mixtures. These interactions, often inhibitions, occur through their metabolism and can be described and quantified using adapted models (Tardif *et al,* 1997).

All these efforts using toxicokinetic models have improved the quantitative understanding of biological monitoring. In recent years, biological monitoring has moved from a fairly descriptive approach to a more mechanistic field, thanks partly to toxicokinetic modeling. This tendency has also been recognised quite early by the authorities. In the description of the work practices used by the BAT committee, simulation studies are one of the three sources of information used to develop BAT values. In the United States, the BEI committee is also very active to include information from simulation studies. This committee has for example published a series of background documents to help users of BEIs. One of them is devoted to toxicokinetic modelling.

Up till now, in the field of biological monitoring toxicokinetic models have mainly been applied to organic chemicals, mostly volatiles,. The toxicokinetic behaviour of these chemicals is relatively easy to simulate and basic information is easily available. In the future toxicokinetic models should be applied also to other groups of chemicals such as metals and metalloids. Of course some work has already been done in this field (Mann *et al*, 1996, Flaherty *et al,* 1995), but models are not as generally available as for solvents. In the future biological monitoring should also benefit from the very active developments of modelling techniques which occur in the fields of risk assessment.

3.6 References

ACGIH, American Conference of Governmental Industrial Hygienists (1999). 1999 TLVs and BEIs. Threshold limit values for chemical substances and physical agents. Biological exposure indices. ACGIH, Cincinnati, OH

Angerer J and Lehnert G (1997). Occupational exposure to methanol. Acta Pharmaol Toxicol 41: 551-556

Cocker J (1996) Human exposure to tetrahydrofurane (personal communication)

d'Alessandro A, Osterloh JD, Chuwers P, Quilan PJ, Kelly TJ and Becker CE (1994). Formate in serum and urine after controlled methanol exposure at the threshold limit value. Environ Health Perspec 102: 178-181

DFG Deutsche Forschungsgemeinschaft (1996). MAK- und BAT-wert-liste 1999. Maximale arbeitzplatzkonzentrationen und biologische arbeitsstofftoleranzwerte. Wiley-VCH, Weinheim, Germany

DFG Deutsche Forschungsgemeinschaft (1999). MAK- und BAT-wert-liste 1999. Maximale arbeitzplatzkonzentrationen und biologische arbeitsstofftoleranzwerte. Wiley-VCH, Weinheim, Germany

Droz PO (1992). Quantification of biological variability, Ann Occup Hyg 36;295-306

Droz PO, Wu MM, Cumberland WG, Berode M(1989). Variability in biological monitoring of solvent exposure. I. Development of a population physiological model. Brit J Ind Med 46: 447-460

Failing A, Knecht U, Woitowitz HJ (1994). Biomonitoring einer standardisierten Tetrahydrofuran-Einwirkung: Daten zur BAT-Wert-Festsetzung. In Arbeitsmedizinische und umweltmedizinische Aspekte zu Altlasten-Bewertung und Bewältigung. Stuttgart, Germany: Bentner Verlag, 1994 pp. 375-376

Flaherty EJO (1995). PBPK modeling for metals. Examples with lead, uranium and chromium. Toxicol Let 82/83: 367-372

Franzblau A, Batterman SA, Zhou N, Stepien CJ, D'Arcy JB, Sargent NE, Gross KB and Schreck RM (1997). Evaluation of methanol and formate in urine as biological exposure indices of methanol exposure. Appl Occup Environ Hyg 12: 367-374

Hattis D, Erdreich L, and Ballew M (1987). Human variability in susceptibility to toxic chemicals- I. A preliminary analysis of pharmacokinetic data from normal volunteers. Risk Anal 7: 415

Heinrich R and Angerer J (1982). Heinrich Occupational chronic exposure to organic solvents. X. Biological monitoring parameters for methanol exposure. Int Arch Occup Environ Health 50: 341-349

Mann S, Droz PO, Vahter M (1996). A physiologically based pharmacokinetic model for arsenic exposure. II Validation and application in humans. Toxicol Appl Pharmacol 140: 471-486

NCHS (1981) National health and nutrition examination survey 1976-1980. National Center for Health Statistics, Hyattsville, Maryland, USA

Nihlen A, Droz PO (1999). Toxicokinetic modeling of methylformate exposure and implications for biological monitoring. Int Arch Occup Environ Health (submitted)

Ogata M and Iwamoto T (1990). Enzymatic assay of formic acid and gas chromatography of methanol for urinary biological monitoring of exposure to methanol. Int Arch Occup Environ Health 62: 227-232

Ong CN, Chia SE, Phoon WH, Tan KT (1991). Biological monitoring of occupational exposure to tetrahydrofuran. Brit J Ind Med 48: 616-621

Tardif R, Charest-Tardif G, Brodeur J, Krishnan K (1997). Physiologically based pharmacokinetic modeling of ternary mixture of alkyl benzenes in rats and humans. Toxicol Appl Pharmacol 144: 120-134

Teramoto K, Wakitani F, Kageyama M, Horiguchi S (1994). Elimination of tetrahydrofuran in man. In Proceedings of the Second Asia-Pacific Symposium on Environmental and Occupational Health, Kobe, Japan 1994, ACGIH Cincinnati OH, pp 177-183

Teramoto K, Yamamoto T, Horiguchi S (1997). Tetrahydrofurane in alveolar air, blood and urine after cessation of exposure. Paper presented at the General Meeting of the Japan Society of Occupational Health, Osaka, Japan

4 DERMAL ABSORPTION FROM PESTICIDE RESIDUES
Data Analysis

MICAELA B.REDDY AND ANNETTE BUNGE

MR: Colorado School of Mines, Golden, CO, USA and CSU.
AB: Colorado State University, Fort Collins, CO, USA.

Abstract: In its regulatory role the United States Environmental Protection Agency is the repository for a large collection of dermal absorption data supplied by pesticide registrants. Many of these studies followed a common procedure measuring dermal absorption *in vivo* into laboratory rats as a function of both the amount of pesticide applied and the exposure time. In this chapter, example registrant data are presented and analyzed. For the 18 pesticides examined in this study, the relationship between systemic absorption and applied dose was different for pesticides that are liquids and those that are solids at skin temperature. For both groups, the amount of pesticide in skin increased proportionally with applied dose. Systemic absorption of liquid pesticides also increased with applied dose. However, for solid pesticides systemic absorption was a weaker function of applied dose and in some cases was independent of applied dose. Finally, a simple method for estimating the maximum systemic absorption using a pesticide's permeability coefficient and water solubility under-estimated the amount of dermal absorption for most doses of many of the pesticides investigated in this study.

4.1 Introduction

Pesticides benefit society in many ways but risk is associated with their use. Besides professional pesticide applicators, farmers and field workers, the general population can be exposed to pesticides in their offices, homes, lawns and swimming pools. Of the routes of human exposure to pesticides (i.e., inhalation, ingestion, and dermal absorption), dermal exposure is the least understood in part due to the limited quantity of pertinent published data.

Most published dermal absorption studies examine exposures to neat chemicals, to large volumes of aqueous solutions, or to residues deposited from acetone. While interesting, results from these investigations are not directly relevant to a typical pesticide exposure in which the active pesticide component and other additives (e.g., surfactants or emulsifiers) contact the skin in a small volume of water. In most cases, the water will evaporate leaving a residue of pesticide and formulation additives on the skin surface.

J. Krüse, H.J.M. Verhaar, and W.K. de Raat (eds.), The Practical Applicability of Toxicokinetic Models in the Risk Assessment of Chemicals, 55-79.

In its regulatory role, the United States Environmental Protection Agency (US EPA) is the repository for a large collection of dermal absorption data supplied by pesticide registrants in compliance with US federal regulations. This database contains almost 300 dermal absorption studies of more than 160 different pesticides (1). Many of these studies followed the Zendzian protocol (2), which prescribes procedural details of *in vivo* rat experiments measuring dermal absorption as a function of both the amount of pesticide applied and the exposure time. Recently, Zendzian (3) reported data collected using the Zendzian protocol for representative pesticides from each of three classifications described as volatile, skin damaging, and neither volatile nor skin damaging.

In this investigation we examine dermal absorption data obtained using the Zendzian protocol for 18 pesticides (Table 1) including data published by Zendzian (3) and data from study summaries provided to us by Zendzian (personal communication). Chemical properties for these pesticides are listed in Table 2. Although many of the 18 studies were performed before the Zendzian protocol was formally issued as a guideline, it is our understanding that all of these studies followed the protocol.

4.2 Background

In addition to the active ingredient, pesticide formulations usually contain inert ingredients that could affect dermal absorption. For example, surfactants are commonly added to improve solution wettability on plant foliage or soil and these might increase dermal absorption by altering the skin barrier or by enlarging the area that the deposited residue covers. It is likely that two pesticide products with the same active ingredient in different formulations might have completely different penetration rates. Unfortunately, in the United States formulation details are protected as confidential business information (CBI) and specifics about formulation ingredients are not generally available.

Experiments studying specific formulations of the 18 pesticides listed in Table 1 were conducted at 3 and sometimes 4 different applied doses, defined as the moles of pesticide applied to skin, M_{app} (nM), per exposed area, A (cm^2). Table 3 lists the applied doses in each study as high (H), medium (M), low (L), and lowest (LL) represented as an apparent film thickness, L_{film} (μm), calculated using Eq. 1.

$$L_{film} = M_{app}\, MW / (A\, \rho) \qquad (1)$$

where MW is molecular weight and ρ is the density of the pesticide film estimated as the density of the pure pesticide. As defined in Eq. 1, L_{film} is the

Table 1. Pesticides Examined in this Study

Pesticide	Report Date[a]	Study MRID[b]	Molecular Formula	Classification
2,4-DP-P-2[E]HE	1/23/97	442293-01	unknown	Unknown
Acetochlor*	10/12/90	417783-01	$C_{14}H_{20}ClNO_2$	Chloroacetanilide
Azinphos-methyl	3/27/92	424527-01	$C_{10}H_{12}N_3O_3PS_2$	Organophosphorous
Diclofop-methyl	5/28/92	423646-01	$C_{16}H_{14}Cl_2O_4$	Phenoxy
Diniconazole	6/18/91	419329-34	$C_{15}H_{17}Cl_2N_3O$	Azole
Disulfoton*	8/30/94	433602-01	$C_8H_{19}O_2PS_3$	Organophosphorous
EPTC	5/9/88	416862-01	$C_9H_{19}NOS$	Thiocarbamate
Imazalil	2/1/93	429134-01	$C_{14}H_{14}Cl_2N_2O$	Azole
Iprodione	10/25/94	435350-03	$C_{13}H_{13}Cl_2N_3O_3$	Dicarboximide
Isoxaflutole	4/25/96	440447-02	$C_{15}H_{12}F_3NO_4S$	Herbicide
Lindane*	1/13/87	400561-07	$C_6H_6Cl_6$	Organochlorine
Metolachlor	8/25/87	418331-02	$C_{15}H_{22}ClNO_2$	Chloroacetanilide
Mevinphos	8/31/93	429338-01	$C_7H_{13}O_6P$	Organophosphorous
Molinate	1/10/91	432841-01	$C_9H_{17}NOS$	Thiocarbamate
Phosmet	3/5/87	401222-01	$C_{11}H_{12}NO_4PS_2$	Organophosphorous
Thiobencarb	8/1/89	412153-11	$C_{12}H_{16}ClNOS$	Thiocarbamate
Tribufos	5/19/92	423500-03	$C_{12}H_{27}OPS_3$	Orthophosphate defoliant
Vinclozlin*	1/3/91	418243-09	$C_{12}H_9Cl_2NO_3$	Dicarboximide

[a] Report date as recorded by US EPA. [b] Report identification number at US EPA.
* Detailed data for these pesticides are presented in this chapter.

theoretical thickness of the pesticide film if the applied dose forms a uniformly thick layer on a flat surface with an area equal to the exposed area.

Usually, dose H was the concentrated formulation, and the other doses were 10-fold dilutions of the next larger dose (e.g., dose M is 1/10th of dose H). The large variations in L_{film} for dose H (from 0.11 to 92 μm) reflect considerable differences in concentrations of active ingredient in the pesticide formulations. Values of L_{film} in Table 3 vary from a low of 0.004 μm for mevinphos to a high of 92 μm for EPTC.

Topographic features of the skin's surface make it likely that L_{film} would need to be larger than about 1 - 10 μm to completely cover the exposed surface. For pesticide exposures like those simulated by the Zendzian protocol, it is likely that the amount of pesticide on the skin often covers only a portion of the exposed skin. Indeed, environmental scanning electron microscopy of a test chemical (4-cyanophenol, a solid at skin temperature) applied to normally hydrated excised human skin at 0.01 mg/cm^2 ($L_{film} \cong 0.1$ μm) using acetone showed chemical-free regions distributed among regions covered by chemical (5).

Table 2. Chemical Properties of Pesticides in this Study (Tomlin, 1997)a.

Pesticide	MW	MP °C	ρ g/cm^3	log$K_{o/w}$	p_{vap} mPa	S_w mg/L
2,4-DP-P-2EHE	347	< 25	unknown[b]	Unknown	unknown	unknown
Acetochlor	270	< 0	1.11	3.03	0.0045[d]	223[d]
Azinphos-methyl	317	73	1.52	2.96	0.001[d]	28[c]
Diclofop-methyl	341	39-41	1.3	4.58	0.25[c]	0.8[c,g]
Diniconazole	326	~ 145	1.32	4.3	4.9[d]	4[d]
Disulfoton	274	< - 25	1.14	3.95	13[d]	25[c]
EPTC	189	< 25	0.95	3.2	0.01[d]	375[d]
Imazalil	297	52.7	1.35	3.82	0.158[d]	180[c]
Iprodione	330	134	1.43[h]	3.0	0.0005[d]	13[c]
Isoxaflutole	359	140	1.59	0.365	0.001[d]	6.2[c]
Lindane	291	113	1.85[f]	3.72[i]	5.6[c]	7.3[d]
Metolachlor	284	- 62.1	1.12	2.9	4.2[d]	488[d]
Mevinphos	224	< 25	1.2	0.127	17[c]	miscible
Molinate	187	< 25	1.06	2.88	746[d]	88[c]
Phosmet	317	72-73	1.03[f]	2.95	0.065[d]	25[d]
Thiobencarb	258	3.3	1.15	3.42	2.93[e]	30[c]
Tribufos	315	< - 25	1.06	3.23	0.71[d]	2.3[c]
Vinclozlin	286	108	1.51	3	0.13[c]	2.6[c]

[a] MW = molecular weight, MP = melting point, ρ = density, $K_{o/w}$ = octanol – water partition coefficient, p_{vap} = vapor pressure, S_w = solubility in water. [b] Estimated as 1.2 for calculation of L_{film}. [c] At 20°C. [d] At 25 °C. [e] At 23 °C. [f] From SPECTRUM website, http://www.speclab.com. [g] At pH = 5.7. [h] For technical grade. [i] From (4).

Similar types of distributions might be expected from dermal exposure to pesticide formulations in which the liquid components evaporate leaving a residue of solid pesticide on the skin surface. The surface distribution of residues might be different for pesticides that are liquids at skin temperature or for formulations in which liquid components do not evaporate.

One would expect that changes in the applied dose or the distribution of a given dose on the skin surface will change the amount of absorption in some situations and produce no change in others. If the applied dose is large enough that chemical completely covers the skin surface for the entire exposure time, the exposed surface is saturated and the absorption rate is maximized. In this case, increasing the applied dose further will not increase the amount that dermally absorbs. But if the amount of chemical on the skin surface is small enough that only a small portion of the exposed area is covered by chemical, then increasing the applied dose will probably increase the area in contact with pesticide and thereby increase the amount of chemical that dermally absorbs.

Table 3. Experimental Details and Selected Results[a]

Pesticide	**Exposure Times, hrs**	**L_{film}, µm**				**S/L**	**Did amount in skin reach a maximum and then decrease?**	**At 10 h, % on skin for all doses**	
		LL	**L**	**M**	**H**			**<50%[d]**	**>50%**
2,4-DP-P-2^{E}HE[e]	0.5,1,2,4,10,24	0.16	0.65	4.1	24	L	No	X[d]	
Acetochlor	0.5,1,2,4,10,24	0.03	0.37	2.4	26	L	No		
Azinphos-methyl	1,4,10	NA	0.006	0.061	0.61	S	No		
Diclofop-methyl	1,2,4,10,24	NA	0.076	0.76	7.7	S?[b]	No	X[d]	
Diniconazole	1,2,4,10,24	NA	0.037	0.38	3.8	S	No		X[c]
Disulfoton	1,4,10	NA	0.0075	0.075	0.75	S	Yes, all doses > 1h	X[d]	
EPTC	1,4,10,24	0.99	2.1	9.5	92	L	Yes, all doses > 1h	X[d]	
Imazalil	0.5,1,2,4,10,24	0.03	0.3	3	30	S	No		
Iprodione	0.5,1,2,4,10,24	NA	0.22	2.2	22	S	No		X
Isoxaflutole	0.5,1,2,4,10,24	NA	0.005	0.05	0.5	S	No		X
Lindane	0.5,1,2,4,10,24	NA	0.11	1.1	11	S	Yes, dose L & M > 4h		
Metolachlor	2,4,10,24	NA	0.089	0.89	8.9	L	Yes, dose L > 4 h		
Mevinphos	6,10,24	NA	0.004	0.021	0.11	L	No	X[d]	
Molinate	4,10,24	NA	0.084	0.84	8.4	L	Yes, all doses > 4h	X[d]	
Phosmet	1,2,4,10,24	NA	0.56	5.1	26	S	No		X[c]
Thiobencarb	1,2,4,10,24	NA	0.045	0.44	4.3	L	Yes, doses L & M > 2h		
Tribufos	1,4,10	NA	0.019	0.095	0.95	L	No		
Vinclozlin	0.5,1,2,4,10	0.013	0.13	1.3	13	S	No		X

[a]NA = not applicable. S/L denotes solid or liquid at skin temperature (~32°C).
[b]The melting point of pure diclofop-methyl is slightly higher than skin temperature (i.e., 39 - 41°C), but the formulation is not pure pesticide and could have a lower melting point.
[c]The percent of applied dose on the skin was not reported, but it probably remained > 50% because the percent in skin and absorbed systemically were low and it is not likely that these pesticides evaporated.
[d]These pesticides were not included in Figures 9 and 10 because the percent of applied dose on the skin at 10 hours was less than 50% for all applied doses.
[e]This pesticide was applied in a vehicle of A260 light mineral oil.
[f]This column notes the doses and exposure times at which the amount in the skin started to decrease due to a decrease in the exposed dose.

However, Reddy (5) showed that absorption from residues partially covering the exposed area with many small piles can be the same as for applied doses that completely cover the exposed area. Thus, one goal of this investigation was to examine the effects of changes in the applied dose on the rate and extent of dermal absorption.

Dermal absorption and evaporation reduce the amount of pesticide remaining on the skin surface. That is, the exposed dose, defined as the amount of pesticide on the skin per exposed area at any time during the exposure, decreases with increased exposure time. If the applied dose is large and dermal absorption and evaporation are slow, the exposed dose will be nearly constant and equal to the applied dose during the entire exposure. However, if dermal absorption or evaporation is rapid, then the exposed dose decreases significantly during the exposure and the rate of continued dermal absorption will be affected. In this case, the exposed dose may not be large enough to saturate the skin surface during the entire exposure time even if the applied dose was large enough to completely cover the skin surface.

Increasing the length of the exposure time will increase the amount of dermal absorption but not always proportionally. After the pesticide formulation is applied to the skin, liquid components of the formulation (e.g., water) will evaporate if their vapor pressure is relatively large. As shown later, dermal absorption does occur during and after liquid components have evaporated. However, the presence of liquid components or the increase in pesticide concentration that occurs as the volume of the remaining liquid components decreases may affect the absorption rate. Furthermore, the rate of dermal absorption usually decreases with exposure time as the skin's capacity for holding chemical is filled. The exposed dose will deviate more from the applied dose with increased exposure time, which also can cause the absorption rate to decrease with exposure time. Clearly, meaningful predictions for dermal absorption of pesticides (and other chemicals with similar types of exposures) will only be possible when the effects of exposure time and applied dose are understood. A goal of this study was to investigate these effects for the 18 pesticides listed in Table 1.

4.3 The Zendzian Protocol

The Zendzian Protocol (2) prescribes the methodology for dermal absorption experiments on young, adult, male laboratory rats (200-250 g). Radiolabeled pesticide is applied to at least 10 cm^2 of the back of a rat that was shaved 24 hrs earlier. The applied volume of a solution does not exceed 10 $\mu L/cm^2$, which is large enough for easy spreading and small enough to minimize the amount that flows to the enclosure. The highest applied dose is typically the concentrated pesticide solution and lower doses are 10-fold dilutions. The solutions are prepared so that the same amount of radiolabeled chemical is applied to the skin irrespective of dose. Thus, the fraction of active ingredient that is radioactive is smallest in the largest dose solution. After application the exposed area is protected by a cover, usually filter paper or gauze, which allows the flow of air without rubbing the surface. If the pesticide is known to evaporate, the cover is impregnated with activated charcoal to prevent additional exposure by vapor inhalation.

Four animals are exposed at each applied dose and exposure time (often including 0.5, 1, 2, 4, 10, and 24 hours). After the exposure ends, the exposed area is washed with soap and water and rinsed, and the animal is then sacrificed. The urine, fecal material, and cage washes are collected and analyzed. The amount of pesticide found on the enclosure and cover, in the skin wash, in the exposed area of the skin, and absorbed through the skin (i.e., found in the carcass, urine, feces, and cage wash) are reported, along with an overall mass balance.

The studies presented here were performed by a variety of different labs. While all used the Zendzian protocol for the basic procedure, the details not precisely specified by the experimental protocol may vary from lab to lab. For example, some labs might apply the pesticide to a circle inside the 10 cm^2 that does not extend to the enclosure and cover while others spread the pesticide over the entire area within the enclosure.

4.4 Results and discussion

Experimental results for all pesticides listed in Table 1 are presented in detail by Reddy (5). Except for one pesticide, acetochlor, the data provided to us (either in (3) or by Zendzian directly) were in the form of the average for four animals with no other statistical information. Here we present results for four pesticides selected as representative of the pesticides in Table 1: acetochlor, disulfoton, lindane and vinclozlin. They were chosen to include examples of a solid (vinclozlin) and a liquid (acetochlor) at skin temperature that did not evaporate, and examples that evaporated rapidly (disulfoton) and slowly (lindane) during the exposure. In most cases, we present the percent of applied dose on the skin surface (i.e., from the skin wash), in the skin at the exposed site, systemically absorbed and recovered as a function of time.

If a pesticide evaporates, the exposed dose on the skin can decrease continuously and significantly during the exposure. Figure 1 shows example results for an evaporating pesticide, disulfoton. Because disulfoton was known to evaporate, activated carbon was included in the cover. As shown in Figure 1a, the percent of applied dose on the enclosure and cover increased with time, indicating that evaporation continued during the entire 10-hour exposure. The percent on the enclosure and cover was smallest for dose H, suggesting that evaporation was more important for the two smaller doses. As indicated in Figure 1e, the percent of applied dose that was

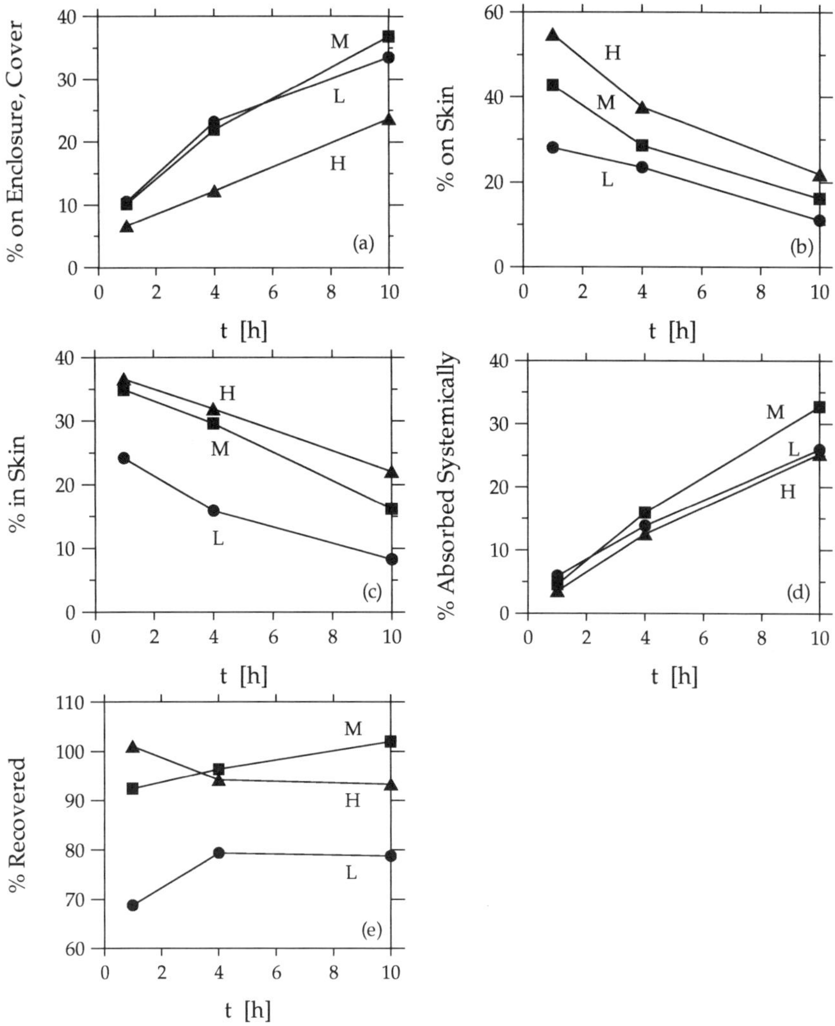

Figure 1. Percent of applied dose of disulfoton (a) on the enclosure and cover, (b) on the skin, (c) in the skin, (d) absorbed systemically and (e) recovered as a function of time for applied doses (●) L, (■) M and (▲) H.

recovered was good (i.e., on average it was > 90%) for doses M and H, but was poorer for dose L.

Figure 1c shows that the amount of disulfoton in the skin reached a maximum at or before one hour, the earliest time for which data were available. For all exposure times studied, the amount in the skin decreased as the amount on the skin decreased. This type of behavior was common when the exposed dose decreased rapidly. By comparing the results from Figure 1b to those in Figure 1a, c and d, it is evident that the amount of pesticide on the skin was decreased by dermal absorption in addition to evaporation. Dermal absorption was responsible for more than half of the pesticide that left the skin surface.

The likelihood of evaporation is indicated by a pesticide's vapor pressure, p_{vap}. For example, p_{vap} for disulfoton is 13 mPa. For 7 of the 18 pesticides listed in Table 2, p_{vap} exceeds 2 mPa. Except for diniconazole and possibly metolachlor, some evaporation was indicated for all pesticides in this group. However, activated carbon covers were not used in the studies of all of these 7 pesticides. When activated carbon was not used, evidence for evaporation was found in other measurements. As an example, for lindane (p_{vap} = 5.6 mPa) the percent of applied dose on the enclosure and cover with no activated carbon was always < 3% (data not shown), but the percent lost in the analysis increased (i.e., the % recovery decreased) continuously over 24 hours (see Figure 2d). For dose L at 24 hours, the percent recovery was less than 60%. Poor recoveries that worsen with time, probably indicate evaporation for pesticides like lindane with p_{vap} greater than 2 mPa.

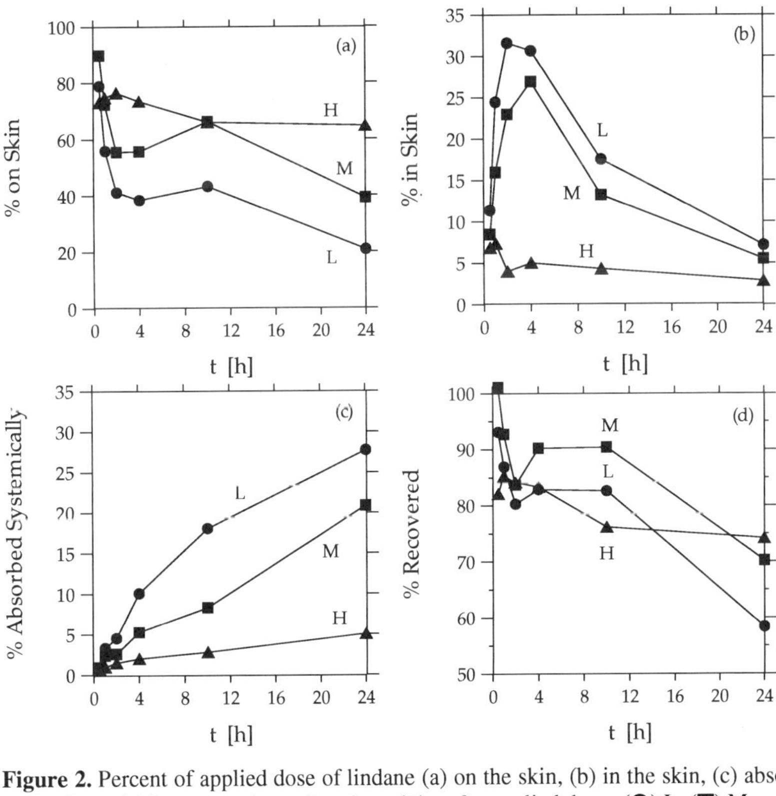

Figure 2. Percent of applied dose of lindane (a) on the skin, (b) in the skin, (c) absorbed systemically and (d) recovered as a function of time for applied doses (●) L, (■) M and (▲) H.

Despite the evaporation of lindane, a solid at skin temperature (MP = 113°C), significant amounts absorbed systemically (Figure 2c). After 24 hours 28% of dose L had absorbed systemically. It has been hypothesized that the majority of dermal absorption of pesticides that are solid at skin temperature will only occur while the liquid solution is present. Clearly, systemic absorption occurred during the entire exposure for lindane. In addition, the amount of lindane in the skin increased between 2 and 4 hours for doses L and M (see Figure 2c). The liquid components in the applied solution would evaporate within about an hour and so dermal absorption into the skin continued from the lindane residue remaining on the skin surface.

The amount of lindane in the skin reached a maximum between 2 and 4 hours, and for doses L and M decreased rapidly after 4 hours as the exposed dose decreased. The amount in skin did not decrease for dose H (Figure 3). This is consistent with the exposed dose at 24 hours, which was 21% for dose L and 39% for dose M, compared to 65% for dose H.

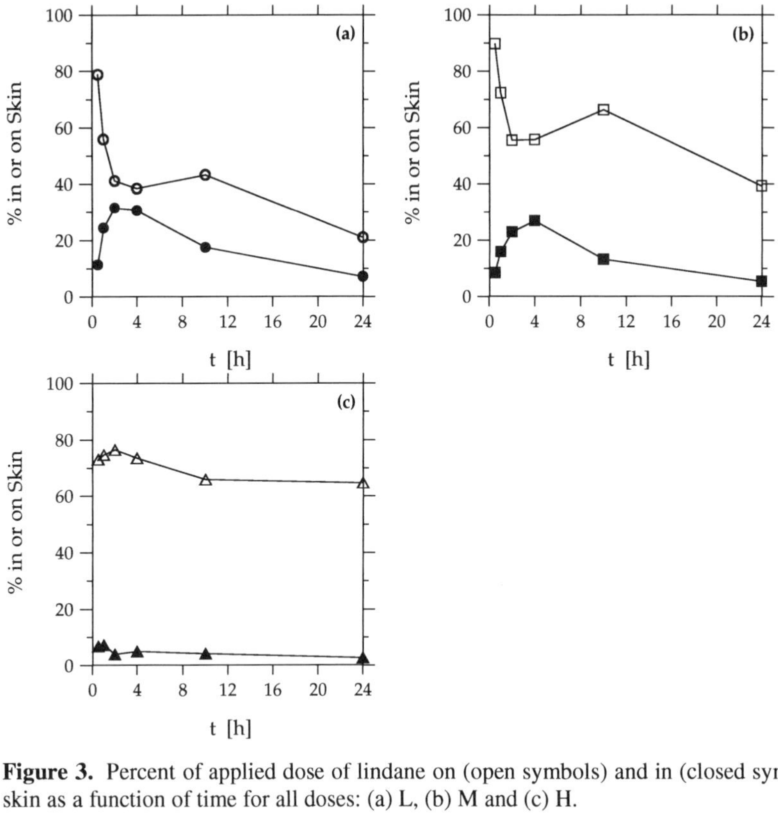

Figure 3. Percent of applied dose of lindane on (open symbols) and in (closed symbols) the skin as a function of time for all doses: (a) L, (b) M and (c) H.

Experimental results for acetochlor are shown in Figure 4. The error bars in Figure 4 represent one standard deviation of a measurement repeated in four rats. To distinguish between applied doses, the error bars increase in width from the lowest to the highest applied dose. Figure 4a shows the percent of applied dose on the cover. The data for dose LL do not include pesticide on the activated carbon filter, which is shown in Figure 4b. The amount of acetochlor on the activated carbon filter was only measured for dose LL because separate experiments (i.e., loss of chemical from a glass slide) suggested that losses by evaporation would only be significant at the smallest dose. Figure 4a shows that up to 20% of the applied dose was found on the cover. The large amount of acetochlor found on the cover probably resulted from a mechanism besides evaporation because it did not increase much with time. For dose LL, the percent on the activated carbon filter increased with exposure time and reached 22% at 24 hours.

There are several reasons that a significant amount of the applied dose may be found on the enclosure and cover. The pesticide might be volatile, the vehicle might migrate to the enclosure over the course of the experiment, or pesticide solution might flow to the enclosing ring during application. When a significant amount of chemical is found on the enclosure and cover, the amount of chemical available for dermal absorption is less than the applied dose indicates.

For acetochlor, the percent of applied dose remaining on the skin decreased for all exposure times due to dermal penetration. The percent in the skin was essentially independent of exposure time, but the percent absorbed systemically increased with time for all doses. In Figures 4a, d and f, there is no significant difference between the doses based on the overlapping error bars. In Figure 4e, the percent absorbed systemically seems to be significantly lower for doses M and H than for doses LL and L. Figure 4d shows that there is probably no statistical difference between the amount of pesticide in the skin at 0.5 and 24 hours.

The exposed dose of acetochlor decreased with increasing exposure time, as shown in Figure 4c. For dose LL at 24 hours, less than 30% of the applied dose remains on the skin. Figure 5 shows, however, that the amount of acetochlor in the skin did not decrease significantly in response to the decreasing exposed dose. Figure 4d shows that the amount of acetochlor in the skin at 24 hours did drop for doses L and LL, but based on the error bars the drop was not significant. Thus, the decrease in the exposed dose probably had a minimal effect on the amount of acetochlor in the skin. For some of the other pesticides, the exposed dose decreased more rapidly.

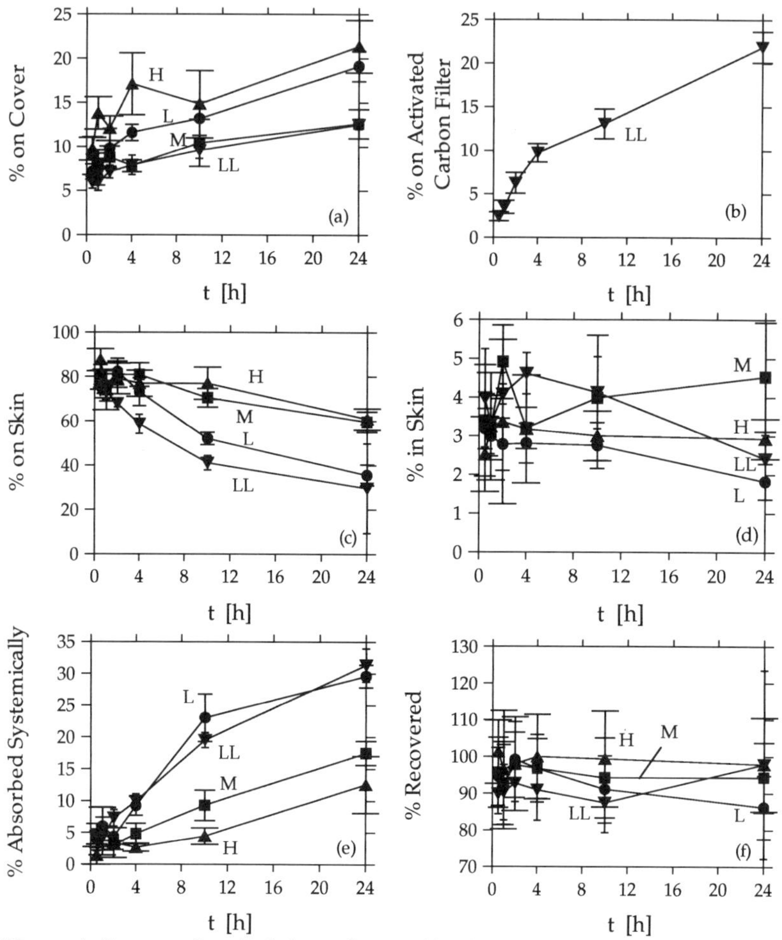

Figure 4. Percent of applied dose of acetochlor (a) on the enclosure and cover, (b) on the activated carbon filter for dose LL, (c) on the skin, (d) in the skin, (e) absorbed systemically and (f) recovered as a function of time for applied doses (▼) LL, (●) L, (■) M and (▲) H.

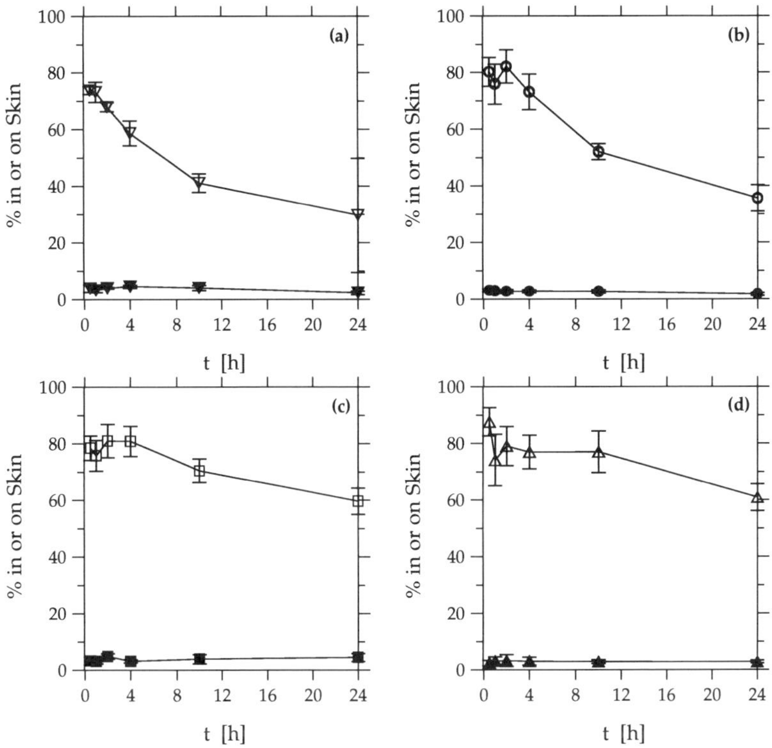

Figure 5. Percent of applied dose of acetochlor on (open symbol) and in (closed symbol) the skin as a function of time for all doses: (a) LL, (b) L, (c) M and (d) H.

The experimental results for vinclozlin shown in Figure 6 do not include the percent recoveries (because they were always greater than 87%), or the percent of applied dose on the enclosure and cover (because these data were not available). In Figure 6a the percent of applied dose on the skin was lowest for dose LL and highest for dose H. The percent in the skin is independent of time (Figure 6b), while the percent absorbed systemically increased with time for all doses. For several data points, the symbol "D" (for detection limit) marks the value that systemic absorption was reported to be less than. For data points marked with D, at least one animal had undetectable systemic absorption, and the detection limit value was used for these animals in the calculation of the mean value. Dose H is most likely to have values below the detection limit because it contains the same amount of radioactivity as the smaller applied doses but the percent absorbed is often smaller for larger doses.

The percent on the skin for vinclozlin decreased by almost 40% for dose LL. However, the amount in the skin did not decrease significantly, as shown in Figure 6b. Apparently, the exposed dose decreased slowly enough or in a way (e.g., the surface area in contact with pesticide did not change)

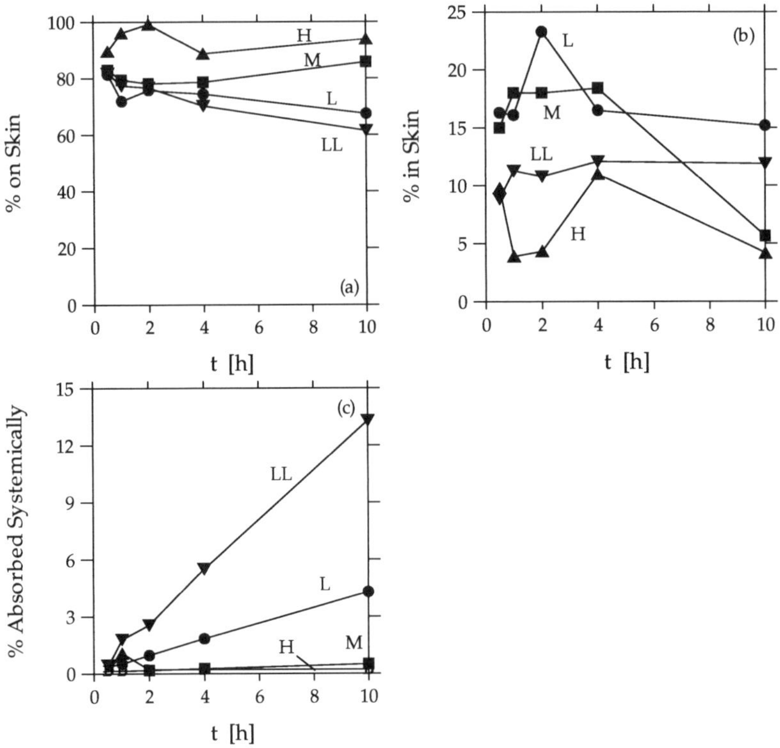

Figure 6. Percent of applied dose of vinclozlin (a) on the skin, (b) in the skin and (c) absorbed systemically as a function of time for applied doses (▼) LL, (●) L, (■) M and (▲) H.

that dermal absorption was not affected. Figure 6 shows that vinclozlin, which is a solid at skin temperature, absorbs into and through the skin after the liquid portion of the formulation has evaporated. For dose LL, the percent of applied dose in the skin remained constant at about 12% between 1 and 24 hours. During that time, systemically absorption increased from 0.4 to 13%.

Comparing the percent in the skin and absorbed systemically as a function of time shows the relative rates of absorption into and through the skin. Some chemicals absorb quickly into the skin but absorb slowly into the bloodstream from the skin. Doses L to H for lindane (L_{film} = 0.11-11 μm) and vinclozlin (L_{film} = 0.13-13 μm) were similar, and lindane (MW = 291, MP = 113°C, $\log K_{o/w}$ = 3.72) and vinclozlin (MW = 286, MP = 108°C, $\log K_{o/w}$ = 3) have similar properties. Comparing Figures 2b to 6b, the percent in the skin was similar for lindane and vinclozlin. After 10 hours, about 5 times more lindane had absorbed systemically than had vinclozlin, even though the exposed dose of lindane decreased more rapidly than it did for vinclozlin. Although lindane and vinclozlin have similar MW, the molar volume of lindane is smaller than vinclozlin (chlorine atoms contribute a smaller molecular volume for their atomic weight compared to carbon and hydrogen). Consequently, lindane probably has a larger diffusion coefficient than vinclozlin, which might explain the observation that in 10 hours more lindane had absorbed than vinclozlin.

When decreases in the exposed dose cause the area in contact with pesticide to decrease, steady state might not occur. In this situation, the amount of pesticide in the skin will increase with time to a maximum value and then may decrease. This was observed for dose L of four of the pesticides listed in Table 1 (i.e., lindane, metolachlor, molinate and thiobencarb), which all reached a maximum amount in the skin within four hours that then decreased significantly. For dose H of these same four pesticides, the amount in the skin increased to a constant value indicating that the amount on the skin was sufficient to apparently saturate the skin. This may or may not coincide with complete coverage of the exposed area. Theoretical calculations (5) have demonstrated that applied doses partly covering the exposed area with many small piles of pesticide can produce as much dermal absorption as a completely covered exposed surface. Thus, it is theoretically possible that decreasing the exposed area by depleting the exposed dose through evaporation or absorption may not always cause the amount of pesticide in the skin to decrease.

Sixteen of the pesticides listed in Table 1 took less than four hours to reach a maximum amount in the skin. If the exposed dose decreased slowly enough, then the time to reach the maximum amount in skin should be related to the lag time for penetration. However, when the exposed dose decreased rapidly, then the maximum might occur more quickly than expected based on the lag time. This is probably what happened for EPTC and disulfoton, which reached a maximum amount in skin at or before one hour, which was the shortest exposure time measured. It is perhaps significant that the two pesticides taking more than four hours to reach a maximum amount in skin had the two largest MW's (i.e., MW is 359 for isoxaflutole and 347 for 2,4-DP-P-2EHE) and perhaps the smallest diffusion coefficients. However, with a similar MW, diclofop-methyl (MW = 341) reached a maximum within one hour.

For diclofop-methyl, the percent in skin reached a constant value before one hour (i.e., for dose L, the percent in skin was 62% at 1 hour and 60% at 10 h) although the exposed dose had decreased in 1 hour to only 25% of the applied dose. The exposed dose decreased rapidly during the first hour of exposure, maybe while the liquid components of the pesticide solution were evaporating. Mevinphos showed a similar pattern. For dose L of mevinphos, the exposed dose decreased to 26% of the applied dose at 6 hours (the shortest exposure time) and 23% at 24 hours, while the percent in skin was

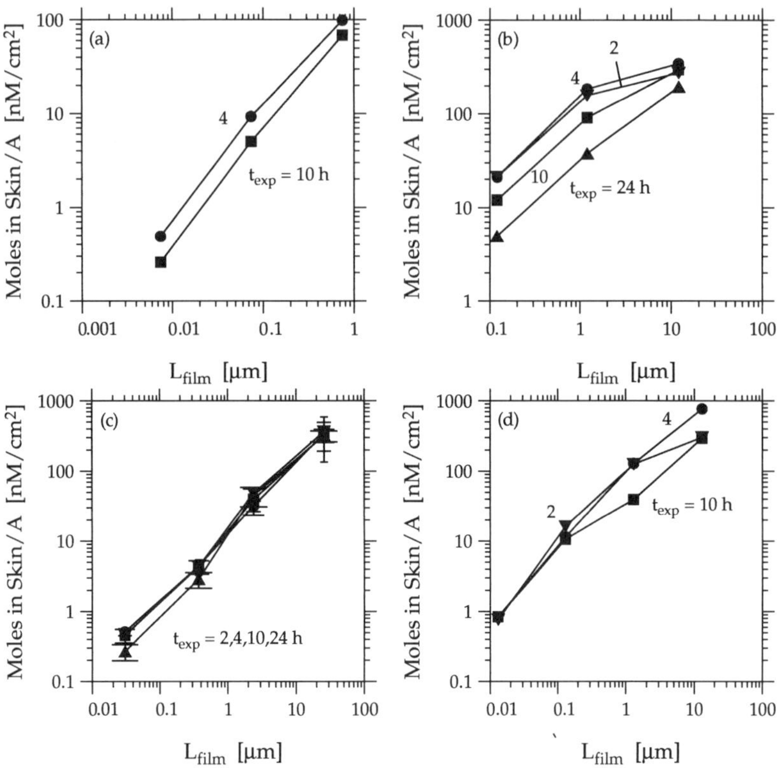

Figure 7. Moles of chemical in the skin as a function of L_{film} for (a) disulfoton, (b) lindane, (c) acetochlor and (d) vinclozlin at (▼) 2, (●) 4, (■) 10 and (▲) 24 hrs.

32% of the applied dose at 6 hours and 30% at 24 hours. Perhaps when the ex posed dose decreased quickly and then became nearly constant, the amount in skin does not decrease after reaching a maximum. For both diclofop-methyl and mevinphos, the maximum amount in the skin was probably smaller than would have been achieved if the exposed dose was the same as the applied dose.

The amount in the skin and absorbed systemically as a function of L_{film} are shown in Figures 7 and 8, respectively, for the four example pesticides to illustrate the effect of applied dose on dermal absorption. In all cases, both the amount in skin and the amount absorbed systemically increased as the applied dose increased. Figures 7a and b show that for the two pesticides with exposed doses that decreased significantly, the amount in the skin was lower for longer exposure times.

Figures 7 and 8 suggest that it might be possible to represent the data using the following equation:

$$M = I\, L_{film}^{\hat{S}} \qquad (2)$$

in which M is the moles per exposed area in the skin or absorbed systemically. Values of $\hat{S}$ and I can be calculated by linearly regressing experimental data to Eq. 3:

$$\log M = \hat{S}\ \log L_{film} + \hat{I} \tag{3}$$

where $\hat{I} = \log I$. If the slope value $\hat{S}$ is approximately one, the moles in the skin or absorbed systemically increased proportionally to dose. If $\hat{S}$ is nearly zero, the moles in the skin or absorbed systemically were independent of applied dose, and further increases in the applied dose caused no increase in the amount absorbed. A value of $\hat{S}$ between zero and one could indicate that dermal absorption is not proportional to applied dose. It could also indicate that for lower applied doses, M increased proportionally to L_{film}, and for higher applied doses M was independent of L_{film}. This might be expected if the amount absorbed was proportional to the surface area in contact with

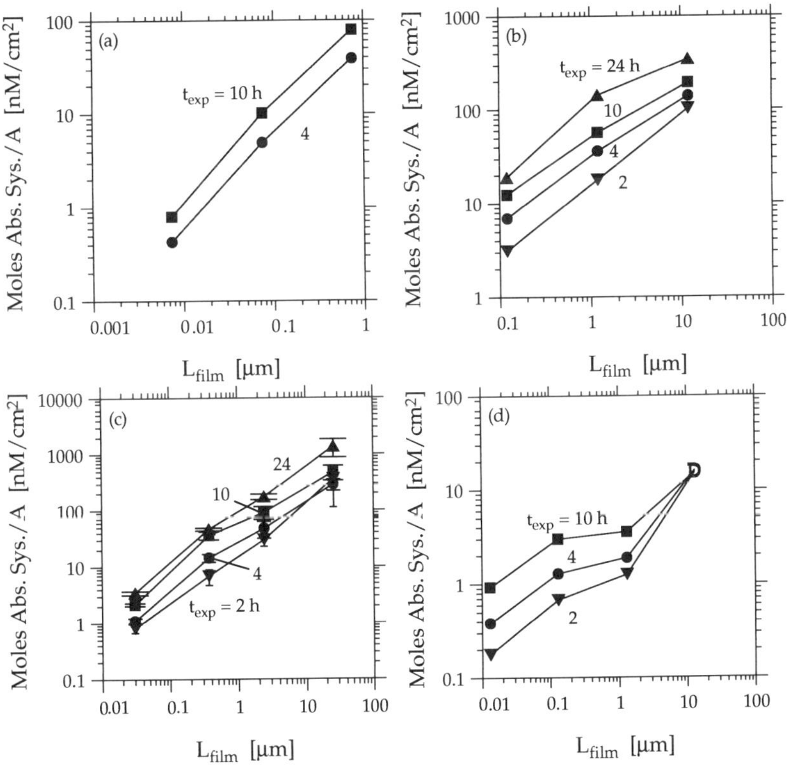

Figure 8. Moles of chemical absorbed systemically as a function of L_{film} for (a) disulfoton, (b) lindane, (c) acetochlor and (d) vinclozlin at (▼) 2, (●) 4, (■) 10 and (▲) 24 hrs.

pesticide for applied doses that were too small to completely cover the skin, and independent of applied dose when the skin is covered enough to saturate. The effect of applied dose was more complicated when the exposed dose changed rapidly with time. For this reason, the data analysis shown in Figure 9 and 10 did not include those pesticides for which the 10-hour exposed dose was less than 50% of the applied dose for all doses (see designation in Table 3). Figure 9 presents the amount in skin and absorbed systemically at 10 hours as a function of L_{film} for four pesticides that are liquids at skin temperature. Figure 10 shows the 10-hour data for eight pesticides that are solid

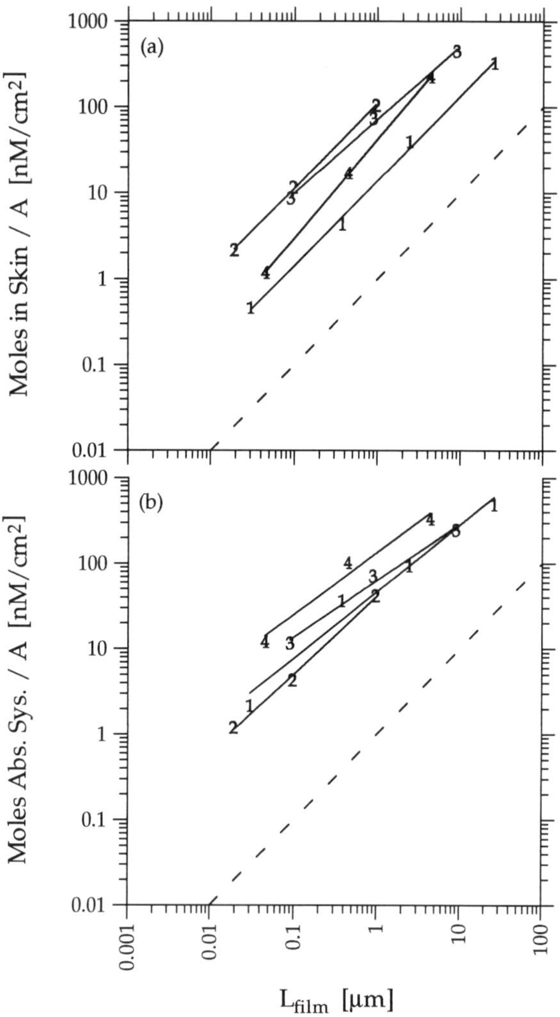

Figure 9. Moles in the skin (a) and moles absorbed systemically (b) as a function of L_{film} for a 10-hour exposure to liquid pesticides: 1 – acetochlor, 2 – tribufos, 3 – metolachlor and 4 – thiobencarb. The dashed line, included as a visual reference, has a slope value of one.

at skin temperature. The 10-hour data were examined because all the studies included a 10-hour exposure, and 10 hours was long enough for the effects of the evaporating vehicle to diminish. In Figures 9 and 10, numbers represent data points and solid lines represent the best-fit unweighted linear regressions to Eq. 3. The dashed line in each plot has a slope of one for visual comparison with the regression lines. Table 4 lists the slope values for the best-fit lines.

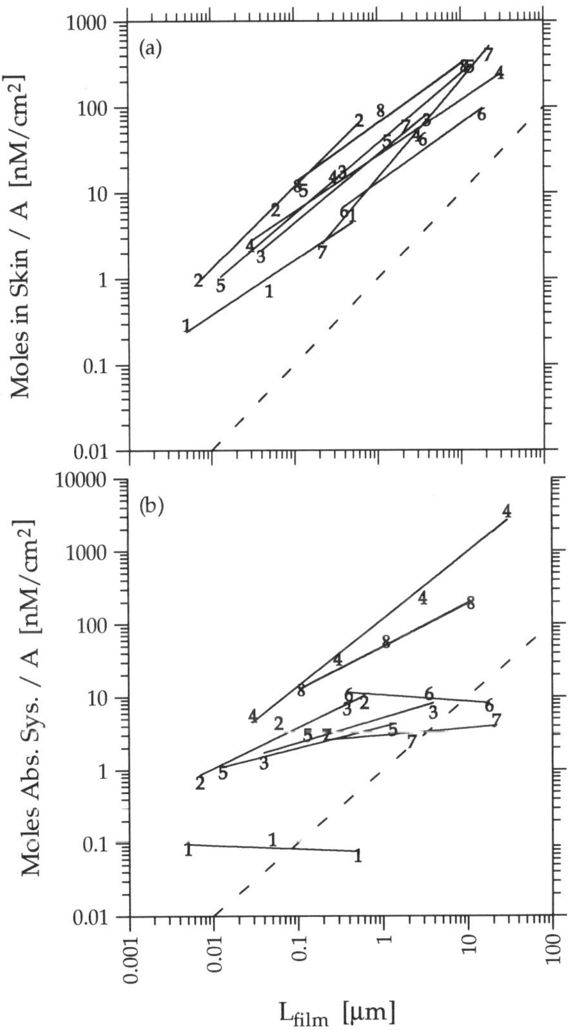

Figure 10. Moles in the skin (a) and moles absorbed systemically (b) as a function of L_{film} for a 10-hour exposure to solid pesticides: 1 – isoxaflutole, 2 – azinphos-methyl, 3 – diniconazole, 4 – imazalil, 5 –vinclozlin, 6 – phosmet, 7 – iprodione and 8 – lindane. The dashed line, included as a visual reference, has a slope value of one.

Unfortunately, only four liquid pesticides met the 50% criterion because, as shown in Table 3, the exposed doses for liquid pesticides tended to be lower than for solid pesticides. Of the pesticides for which the exposed dose was greater than 50% at 10 hours, all five were solids. Of the pesticides for which all the exposed doses at 10 hours were less than 50%, five out of six were liquid pesticides.

As indicated in Table 4, $\hat{S}$ for the amount in skin was typically greater than or equal to $\hat{S}$ for the amount absorbed systemically. Imazalil is the notable exception. For imazalil, values of $\hat{S}$ for the amount in the skin were 0.7 – 0.8 for all exposure times, but for the amount absorbed systemically $\hat{S}$ increased with exposure time from 0.5 at 4 hours to 0.9 at 24 hours. These observations are consistent with a chemical that damages the skin. Exposure to imazalil has caused some sensitive test animals to experience contact dermatitis (6). Also, some formulations of imazalil have been given the US EPA toxicity classification II, indicating that it can cause severe skin irritation within 72 hours (7).

Table 4. Regression Coefficients for Moles of Pesticide in the Skin and Absorbed Systemically as a Function of L_{film} for the 10-Hour Exposure.

S / L[a]	Pesticide	$\log K_{o/w}$ [b]	Range of L_{film}, μm	$\hat{S}$	
				in skin	abs. sys.
L	acetochlor	3.03	0.027-26	1.1	0.87
L	metolachlor	2.9	0.089-8.9	0.86	0.54
L	thiobencarb	3.42	0.045-4.3	1.1	0.72
L	tribufos	3.23	0.019-0.95	0.99	0.91
S	azinphos-methyl	2.96	0.006-0.61	0.93	0.55
S	diniconazole	4.3	0.037-3.8	0.79	0.34
S	imazalil	3.82	0.03-30	0.65	0.92
S	iprodione	3.0	0.22-22	1.1	0.098
S	isoxaflutole	0.365	0.005-0.5	0.64	-0.049
S	lindane	3.72	0.11-11	0.70	0.59
S	phosmet	2.95	0.56-26	0.69	-0.086
S	vinclozlin	3	0.013-13	0.82 (0.84)[c]	(0.29)[c]

[a] S / L denotes solid or liquid at skin temperature (~ 32°C).

[b] See Table 2 for references.

[c] Calculated using data for doses LL, L, and M because the amount absorbed systemically for dose H was below the detection limit.

For both solid and liquid pesticides, the amount in the skin increased with L_{film}. This indicates that for doses lower than dose H, the skin could not have been completely covered with pesticide. To clearly identify the applied dose that saturates the skin, data for at least two larger doses and two smaller doses are needed. Dose H might or might not have been completely covered by pesticide.

Figures 9 and 10 indicate that there could be a difference in the effect of applied dose on dermal absorption for solid and liquid pesticides. In fact, for three of the solid pesticides (i.e., iprodione, isoxaflutole, and phosmet) the amount absorbed systemically was essentially independent of L_{film} but the amount in the skin was almost proportional to L_{film}. For liquid pesticides, the slope values for the moles absorbed systemically tend to be only slightly smaller than slope values for the moles of pesticide in the skin. One possible explanation for this was examined theoretically by Reddy (5), who showed that the flux through the skin can reach a maximum value at smaller applied doses than the amount in the skin when chemical is distributed spatially on skin in piles with dimensions that are comparable to or smaller than the apparent thickness of the sc. The data shown in Figures 9 and 10 suggest that the distribution of solid and liquid pesticide residues on the skin surface might be different.

To assess the risk associated with pesticide use, it is necessary to estimate the amount of dermal absorption that might occur during an exposure. Lacking other data, some investigators have proposed estimating dermal absorption using predicted values of a pesticide's permeability coefficient through skin from water ($P_{skin,w}$) combined with its water solubility (S_w). Since the thermodynamic activity of a saturated aqueous solution is the same as for the pure compound, the maximum flux from water (= $P_{skin,w}\ S_w$) should also represent the flux from a pure compound that completely covers the exposed area when there is no mass transfer resistance between the compound and skin. Consequently, for a given exposure time t_{exp}, the maximum amount absorbed systemically (M_{max}) could be estimated as:

$$M_{max} \approx P_{skin,w}\ S_w \left(t_{exp} - t_{lag}\right) \qquad (4)$$

in which t_{lag} is the lag time for diffusion across skin. Table 5 lists estimated values of $P_{skin,w}$ calculated for 16 of the pesticides listed in Table 1 using one of many possible correlations based on octanol-water partitioning ($K_{o/w}$) and MW (8,9):

$$\log P_{skin,w}\,(\mathrm{cm/hr}) = -2.72 + 0.71\ \log K_{o/w} - 0.0061\ \mathrm{MW} \qquad (5)$$

Table 5. Estimated Values of Maximum Absorption Compared to Experimental Values*

Pesticide[§]	$P_{skin,w}$ cm/hr	M_{max} in 10 hrs, μg/cm²	3 x M_{max} in 10 hrs, μg/cm²	Experimental Systemic Absorption in 10 hrs, μg/cm²			
				LL	L	M	H
acetochlor	0.0061	14	42	0.59	9.8	25	130
azinphos-methyl	0.0028	0.79	2.4	NA	0.22	1.4	2.7
diclofop-methyl	0.028	0.23	0.69	NA	0.89	15	78
diniconazole	0.022	0.88	2.6	NA	0.41	2.2	2.0
"	"	"	"	[a] NA	[a] 0.17	[a] 0.40	[a] 2.0
disulfoton	0.026	6.5	19	NA	0.22	2.8	21
EPTC	0.025	94	280	4.3	6.6	40	430
imazalil	0.015	27	81	1.7	9.8	68	1000
iprodione	0.0025	0.32	0.96	NA	1.0	0.80	1.5
isoxaflutole	0.000022	0.0014	0.0042	NA	0.030	0.040	0.024
Lindane	0.014	0.99	3.0	NA	3.6	17	56
Metolachlor	0.0040	20	60	NA	3.3	20	70
Molinate	0.015	13	39	NA	2.1	34	310
Phosmet	0.0028	0.69	2.1	NA	3.4	3.5	2.4
Thiobencarb	0.014	4.1	12	NA	3.1	26	85
Tribufos	0.0045	0.10	0.30	NA	0.38	1.4	13
Vinclozlin	0.0046	0.12	0.36	0.27	0.86	1.0	< 4.4

* From reference (5).

§ 2,4-DP-P-2EHE was not included because $K_{o/w}$ was unknown and mevinphos was not included because it does not have a solubility limit in water.

[a]Data from US EPA MRID 419329-33 (12/3/90) supplied by reference (1).

In addition, Table 5 provides values of M_{max} for a 10-hour exposure estimated using Eq. (4) and assuming $t_{lag} = 0$.

As shown in Table 5, M_{max} under-estimated the experimental systemic absorption for most doses of many of the pesticides. Eq. (4) was derived from data for human skin, which is reported to be less permeable than rat skin, perhaps by a factor of 2 or 3 (10). Table 5 also lists 3 x M_{max}, which is still smaller than many of the experimental measurements.

4.5 Conclusions

The amount of pesticide absorption increased with exposure time. For all but two of the pesticides (isoxaflutole and 2,4-DP-P-2EHE), the amount of

chemical in the skin reached a maximum within 4 hours of exposure. For all 18 pesticides, the cumulative amount absorbed systemically increased for all exposure times up to 24 hours. Significantly, dermal absorption continued even after the liquid components of the applied solution had evaporated.
When either evaporation or dermal absorption was significant, the exposed dose remaining on the skin surface decreased enough to affect dermal absorption. For six pesticides (disulfoton, EPTC, lindane, metolachlor, molinate, and thiobencarb), the effects of the decreasing exposed dose were apparent in that the amount in the skin increased, reached a maximum, and then decreased with time. For two pesticides (diclofop-methyl and mevinphos), the exposed dose decreased rapidly to less than 35% of the applied dose, and the amount in the skin reached a constant that was probably related to the exposed dose rather than the applied dose.
The relationship between applied dose and dermal absorption was more complicated when the exposed dose decreased significantly during the exposure from either evaporation or dermal absorption. Consequently, we examined the effect of applied dose on data for 12 of the 18 pesticides, excluding pesticides that had less than 50% of the applied dose remaining on the skin for all doses at 10 hours. This analysis showed a difference between solid and liquid pesticides. For pesticides with melting points below skin temperature (i.e., liquids), both the amount of pesticide in the skin and the amount absorbed systemically increased almost proportionally with applied dose. For pesticides with melting points above skin temperature (i.e., solids), the amount in the skin increased almost proportionally to the applied dose, but the amount absorbed systemically was less than proportional to applied dose for some pesticides and was independent of applied dose for others. Significantly, a simple method for estimating the maximum amount of pesticide absorbed systemically using a pesticide's permeability coefficient and water solubility under-estimated the amount of dermal absorption for most doses of many of the pesticides investigated in this study.

Acknowledgements

This work was supported in part by the US Environmental Protection Agency (CR824053 and PR-DC-99-01933/2W9F09).

Notation

A	=	surface area of chemical exposure
I	=	coefficient of an equation that can be used to describe data for the amount in the skin or the amount absorbed systemically
$\hat{I}$	=	intercept of the best-fit line for the log-log plot of the amount in the skin or absorbed systemically as a function of L_{film}

$K_{o/w}$ = octanol – water partition coefficient
L_{film} = theoretical thickness of the applied dose if it formed a uniformly thick layer on a flat surface with an area equal to the exposed area
M = variable in regression equation representing either the moles per area in skin or absorbed systemically
M_{app} = moles of pesticide applied to the skin
M_{max} = estimated maximum amount of pesticide absorbed systemically for an exposure of time t_{exp}
MP = melting point
MW = molecular weight
$P_{skin,w}$ = permeability coefficient for a chemical penetrating skin from an aqueous solution
p_{vap} = vapor pressure
$\hat{S}$ = slope of the best-fit line for the log-log plot of the amount in the skin or absorbed systemically as a function of L_{film}
S_w = water solubility
t_{exp} = exposure time
t_{lag} = lag time

GREEK

ρ = density of a pure pesticide

4.6 References

1. Zendzian, R.P. personal communication, 2000.
2. Zendzian, R.P. Pesticide Assessment Guidelines. Subdivision F, Hazard Evaluation, Human and Domestic Animals: Dermal Absorption of Pesticides, Office of Pesticide Programs, US Environmental Protection Agency, Washington, DC, 1994.
3. Zendzian, R.P. Dermal absorption of pesticides in the rat. Am Ind Hyg Assoc J 2000; 61.
4. Hansch, C., Leo, A., Hoekman, D., Exploring QSAR. Hydrophobic, electronic, and steric constants. Washington, DC: American Chemical Society, 1995.
5. Reddy, M.B. Examining Issues in Percutaneous Transport Using Mathematical Models. Ph.D. Thesis, Colorado School of Mines, Golden, CO, 2000.
6. EXTOXNET. Pesticide information profile: Imazalil. , Vol. 1999
7. Tomlin, C., ed. The Pesticide Manual, England: The British Crop Protection Council, 1997.
8. Potts, R.O., Guy, R.H. Predicting skin permeability. Pharm Res 1992; 9:663-9.
9. Bunge, A.L., McDougal, J.N. "Dermal uptake." In Exposure to Contaminants in Drinking Water: Estimating Uptake through the Skin and by Inhalation/, S. Olin, ed. Boca Raton, FL: CRC Press, 1999; 137-81.
10. Vecchia, B.E. Estimating the Dermally Absorbed Dose from Chemical Exposure: Data Analysis, Parameter Estimation, and Sensitivity to Parameter Uncertainties. M.S. Thesis, Colorado School of Mines, Golden, CO, 1997.

5 INTER-SPECIES PHARMACOKINETIC COMPARISON OF ORGANIC ACID HERBICIDES. IS THE DOG A RELEVANT SPECIES FOR EVALUATION OF HUMAN HEALTH RISK?

CHARLES TIMCHALK[1], RICHARD NOLAN[2], RICHARD BILLINGTON[2] AND DAVID L. EISENBRANDT[2]

[1]*Battelle, Pacific NW Div.Molecular Biosciences, Chemical Dosimetry Group Battelle Boulevard, Richland, WA., U.S.A.*
[2]*Dow AgroSciences, 9550 Zionsville Rd,.Indianapolis, IN, U.S.A.*

Abstract: 3,5,6-Trichloro-2-pyridinyloxyacetic acid (triclopyr) and 2,4-dichlorophenoxyacetic acid (2,4-D) are widely utilized herbicides that have undergone extensive toxicity and pharmacokinetic analysis. Based on this large data-base, the dog appears to exhibit the lowest No-Observed-Effect Levels (NOEL) relative to other species that have undergone toxicological evaluation. It is proposed that this unique sensitivity of the dog to organic acid herbicides is primarily due to the dog's low capacity, relative to other species (including humans), to excrete organic acids. The excretion of organic acids, like triclopyr and 2,4-D, in the kidney is the net result of filtration, secretion and reabsorption processes. Although renal clearance mechanisms for organic acids are ubiquitous in mammalian species there are qualitative differences between species that account for observed discrepancies in clearance capacity. The pharmacokinetics and metabolism of triclopyr and 2,4-D are fairly consistent across species (including the dog), these herbicides are rapidly absorbed following oral administration and quickly cleared from the body into the urine predominantly unmetabolized. Allometric parameter scaling was used to compare the triclopyr and 2,4-D pharmacokinetic parameters across species. The results of this analysis clearly illustrated the decreased capacity of the dog to effectively clear these organic acids relative to other species, including humans. In addition, this decreased clearance capacity of the dog is not compound specific, but is associated with organic acids that share common pharmacokinetic properties: as (1) extensive but reversible plasma protein-binding, (2) weak acids that are highly ionized at physiological pH, (3) limited metabolism of the parent acid, and (4) urinary excretion primarily involving a saturable, active secretion. The most likely mechanism responsible for the lower clearance in the dog, is a low capacity to actively secrete organic acids by the kidney. Other potential mechanisms for the lower clearance such as increased reabsorption from the tubules can not be excluded. This comparative species evaluation of the pharmacokinetics and renal clearance of triclopyr and 2,4-D questions the relevance of using dog toxicity data for the extrapolation of human health risk for these organic acids. Based on the lack of a pharmacokinetic concordance between the dog and other mammalian species it is suggested that the dog is not a reasonable surrogate for humans. Therefore, from a risk assessment perspective, it would seem prudent to utilize toxicity data from other species (e.g. rodents) for extrapolation of human health risk for these organic acid herbicides.

J. Krüse, H.J.M. Verhaar, and W.K. de Raat (eds.), The Practical Applicability of Toxicokinetic Models in the Risk Assessment of Chemicals, 79-107.

5.1 Background

In the United States and within the European Community agricultural chemicals are subjected to a rigorous registration process. A cornerstone of this evaluation is the need to provide the regulatory authorities with a comprehensive toxicological data package that includes acute, sub-chronic, and chronic toxicity evaluation in multiple laboratory species including dogs. Within the review process the regulatory agencies access the adequacy and completeness of the registrant's data set and utilize the data to establish a reference dose (RfD) or an Allowable Occupational Exposure Limit (AOEL) for the chemical. In general, the RfD or AOEL is set based on the existing data at that time utilizing the lowest No-Observed-Effect-Level (NOEL) and appropriate uncertainty factors to account for inter-species extrapolation and intra-species variability.

In this manuscript we will present two examples in which comparative pharmacokinetic data were used to provide scientific justification for not using the NOEL from the dog (lowest NOEL) to establish an RfD or AOEL for human exposure. The herbicides of interest were 3,5,6-trichloro-2-pyridinyloxyacetic acid (triclopyr) and 2,4-dichlorophenoxyacetic acid (2,4-D), which were both recently under review by the U.S. EPA and European regulatory authorities, respectively. In these particular cases a similar scientific approach was used for both chemicals to address the concerns of regulators in the U.S. and in Europe. The primary technical approach entailed the following: 1) to provide strong scientific evidence supporting the hypothesis that for these organic acids the dog was not a relevant species for extrapolation of risk to humans; 2) to demonstrate that the low dose response observed in the dog was a physiological response associated with organic acids competing for the same active transport system; and 3) to conduct appropriate mode of action studies that provide some understanding of the mechanism for renal organic acid clearance in the dog.

The overall objectives of this manuscript are to present the technical arguments that were used to address the question of the dog relevancy, and to illustrate how the results impacted the regulatory process for both triclopyr and 2,4-D.

The organic acids triclopyr and 2,4-D are widely utilized chlorinated pyrinyloxy- and phenoxyacetic acid herbicide, respectively. These herbicides are used to control a wide variety of broad leaf and woody plants and share similar chemistry, herbicidal action and pharmacokinetic properties in several mammalian species including humans (Arnold and Beasley, 1989; Gehring and Betso, 1978; Munro *et. al.*, 1992; Timchalk, *et al.*, 1990; Timchalk and Nolan, 1997; Carmichael *et al.*, 1989). The chemical structure of both triclopyr and 2,4-D are presented in Figure 1.

Triclopyr (3,5,6-trichloro -2-pyridinyloxyacetic acid)

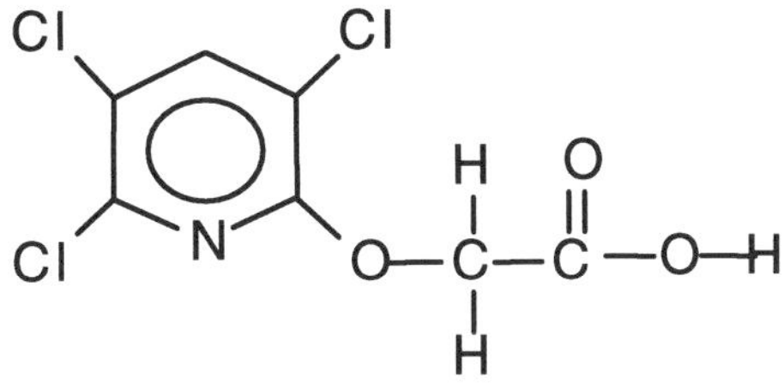

2,4-D (dichlorophenoxyacetic acid)

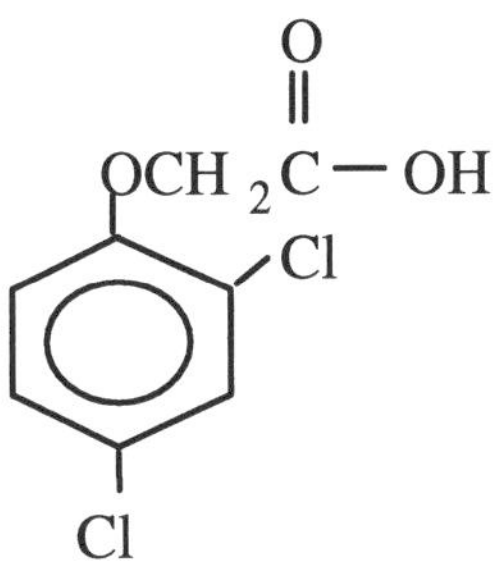

Figure 1. Chemical structure of Triclopyr, 3,5,6-trichloro-2-pyrinyloxyacetic acid; and 2,4-D, 2,4-dichlorophenoxyacetic acid.

5.2 Toxicology Background

Triclopyr has been extensively evaluated for acute, sub-chronic and chronic toxicity in both rodents (mice and rats) and dogs. Triclopyr has a low acute toxicity with an oral LD_{50} in rats of 713 mg/kg (Worthing, 1987). Sub-chronic (13 week) dietary administration of 5 - 250 mg/kg/day of triclopyr resulted in slight degeneration of the descending proximal tubules (S3 segment) of the kidneys in rats given 20 mg/kg/day or more (Landry *et al.*, 1985). Chronic dietary administration to rats resulted in no tumorigenic response and no adverse effects (NOEL) were observed in rats treated with 3 mg triclopyr/kg/day (Eisenbrandt *et al.*, 1988; EPA, 1995). A 1-year chronic dietary study was conducted in the dog at doses of 0, 0.5, 2.5 and 5 mg/kg/day; the kidney was identified as a target organ (1988; unpublished report of the Dow Chemical Co., Midland, MI). The NOEL for the chronic dog study was 0.5 mg/kg/day. The kidney effects observed at 2.5 and 5 mg/kg/day were characterized by a slight reduction in phenolsulfonphthalein (PSP) excretion, slight increase in blood urea nitrogen (BUN) and creatinine, and of a pigment normally occurring in the proximal tubules of the kidneys. These minor changes were interpreted to be a reversible physiological adaptation associated with excretion of the test material. Therefore, the no-observed-adverse-effect level (NOAEL) was considered to be 5 mg/kg/day, which is 10 fold higher that the observed NOEL in the same study. The 0.5 mg/kg NOEL for triclopyr cited by the EPA (1995) for the dog is consistently lower than for the rat.

The phenoxyacetic acid 2,4-D has likewise been extensively tested in animals for acute, sub-chronic and chronic toxicity and the reader is referred to the comprehensive review of Munro *et al.*, (1992) on the safety evaluation of 2,4-D. This phenoxyacetic acid herbicide demonstrates a low acute toxicity with LD_{50s} ranging from ~360 – 700 mg/kg in rats, mice, chickens and guinea-pigs (Rowe and Hymans, 1954; Gorzinski *et al.*, 1987). However, in dogs the acute LD_{50} is reported to range from 24 – 250 mg/kg (Rowe and Hymans, 1954; Dlagard-Mikkelsen and Poulsen, 1962). Overall, the two main target organs for 2,4-D toxicity are the kidney and the thyroid (rat only) with kidneys being the most sensitive (Munroe *et al.*, 1992). Sub-chronic dietary administration of 2,4-D at doses ranging from 15 – 150 mg/kg/day (13-weeks) resulted in treatment-related cytoplasmic alterations in the renal proximal tubules of most rats given 60 mg/kg/day or higher (Gorzinski *et al.*, 1987). A dose-related degenerative change was identified in the descending proximal renal tubules of all male rats given 60 mg/kg/day or higher and in some rats given the 15 mg/kg/day dose. The NOEL in this study was determined to be less than 15 mg/kg/day. Charles *et al.* (1996a) evaluated the chronic toxicity and oncogenicity of 2,4-D in both mice and rats. They reported no oncogenic effect and the chronic toxicity paralleled the sub-chronic findings, and established a NOEL of 5 mg/kg/day. Sub-chronic and chronic toxicity evaluation of 2,4-D was also conducted in dogs comparing the parent acid with the salt and ester formulations (Charles *et al.*, 1996b). In the 1-year chronic study, dogs were administered doses of 0, 1, 5 and 7.5 mg/kg/day. The kidney was identified as a target organ and minor treatment related increases in BUN and creatinine were noted. The NOEL for the chronic dog study was determined to be 1 mg/kg/day.

Overall, these findings with triclopyr and 2,4-D are consistent with each other and with previous reports that indicated the dog is particularly susceptible (lower NOEL) to the effects of organic acids relative to other animal species (Arnold and Beasley, 1989; Gehring and Betso, 1978).

5.3 Hypothesis

It is proposed that the unique sensitivity of the dog to the renal effects of organic acids, such as triclopyr and 2,4-D, are primarily due to the dog's low capacity, relative to other species (including humans), to excrete organic acids. It is likewise proposed that this greater sensitivity of the dog will be observed for various organic acids that share common pharmacokinetic properties: including (1) extensive but reversible plasma protein-binding, (2) weak acids that are highly ionized at physiological pH, (3) limited metabolism of the parent acid, and (4) urinary excretion primarily involving a saturable, active secretion.

5.4 Approach

A strategy was developed to adequately support this hypothesis, and provide a rational scientific argument for not utilizing the dog toxicity data for human risk assessment to both triclopyr and 2,4-D. The cornerstone of the strategy involved obtaining comparative species pharmacokinetic data for both triclopyr and 2,4-D. This was accomplished through experimentation and by evaluating the extensive pharmacokinetic data-base that is available on these organic acids. The following key questions were addressed:

- Is the clearance of triclopyr and 2,4-D slower in the dog relative to other species including humans?
- How are organic acids cleared in the kidneys of dogs and excreted in the urine?
- Are renal functional changes a toxicological response or a physiological adaptation associated with the excretion of organic acids?
- What potential mechanism(s) may be responsible for the reduced elimination of organic acids in the dog?
- Is the dog toxicity data obtained with either triclopyr or 2,4-D of any relevance for the extrapolation of human health risk?

Comparative Pharmacokinetics. Triclopyr and 2,4-D are organic acids and both are well absorbed orally, extensively bound to plasma proteins (reversible), have a similar tissue distribution profile, undergo limited metabolism and are eliminated quickly from the body primarily unchanged in the urine by active saturable renal transport (Gehring and Betso, 1978; Arnold and Beasley, 1989; Timchalk and Nolan, 1997; Timchalk *et al.*, 1990; Gorzinski *et al.*, 1987). The mechanisms responsible for the renal clearance of triclopyr and 2,4-D have been investigated in several species. Both organic acids have been shown to effectively compete with other organic acids (i.e. PAH, PSP) for a common renal transport system (Koschier *et al.*, 1978; Berndt and Koschier, 1973; Erne and Sperber, 1974; Timchalk *et al.*, 1997). This hypothesis is consistent with studies that have repeatedly demonstrated a decreased renal clearance when these organic acids were co-administered (Russel *et al.*, 1989; 1987a,b, Mann *et al.*, 1991; Foreman, 1984; Weiner, 1974). This mechanism of renal clearance for 2,4-D and triclopyr is consistent with that of other phenoxyacetic acids (Hook *et al.*, 1974; Berndt and Koschier, 1973; Braunlich *et al.*, 1989). It has been suggested that the observed dose-dependent non-linear pharmacokinetics of triclopyr and 2,4-D are primarily due to the saturation of this renal secretory transport system (Gehring and Betso, 1978; Arnold and Beasley, 1989; Timchalk *et al.*, 1990; Timchalk and Nolan, 1997).

Various aspects of the pharmacokinetics and metabolism of triclopyr and 2,4-D have been studied in numerous species including: mice, rats, dogs, pigs, calves, monkeys and humans (Arnold and Beasley, 1989; Erne, 1966; Gehring and Betso, 1978; Gorzinski *et al.*, 1987; Griffin *et al.*, 1997; Grizzle *et al.*, 1995; Orberg, 1980; Pelletier *et al.*, 1989; Sauerhoff *et al.*, 1977; Kim *et al.*, 1994; Eiseman, 1984; Smith *et al.*, 1980; Timchalk *et al*, 1990; Timchalk and Nolan, 1997). Both triclopyr and 2,4-D have demonstrated dose-dependent non-linear pharmacokinetics in multiple species (Eiseman, 1984; Gorzinzki *et al.*, 1987; Smith *et al.*, 1980; Kim *et al.*, 1995; Timchalk *et al.*, 1990; Timchalk and Nolan, 1997). To facilitate understanding the toxicological implications of species differences in pharmacokinetics of both triclopyr and 2,4-D, relevant parameters were obtained or calculated from the literature. Three parameters that were of particular importance for the comparative species pharmacokinetics evaluation were the volume of distribution (Vd), renal clearance (Clr), and plasma half-life ($t_{1/2}$). Due to dose-dependent non-linear pharmacokinetics, these parameters were compared across species at dose levels were the kinetics were essentially first order.

The results of the comparative species pharamacokinetic analysis for triclopyr and 2,4-D are presented in Table 1 and 2, respectively. The appar-ent Vd for both triclopyr and 2,4-D increase as a function of body weight and was only slightly larger than the blood volume suggesting that both chemicals primarily resided in the blood and extracellular water. In the dog, the renal Clr of triclopyr (0.95 mL hr^{-1} kg^{-1}) was 17 to 78 fold lower than that observed in the mice, rat, monkey, pig, calf and human (range 17 to 78 mL hr^{-1} kg^{-1}). For triclopyr the plasma $t_{1/2}$ ranged from 3.4 – 25 hr in rat, dog,

Table 1. Selected comparative species triclopyr pharmacokinetic parameters calculated from the literature.

Parameters	Units	Rat[a]	Monkey[b]	Dog[b]	Human[c]
Body weight (Bdwt)	kg	0.2	5.7	8.6	71
Dose	mg kg^{-1}	3	30	0.5	0.1
Renal clearance (Clr)	mL hr^{-1}	29.4	11.8	273	3120
Renal clearance (Clr)[d]	mL hr^{-1} kg^{-1}	147	48	1.4	44
Volume distribution (Vd)	L	0.01	0.72	1.4	12.35
Plasma half-life ($t_{1/2}$)	hr	3.4	6.3	25	5

[a]Timchalk *et al.* (1990); [b]Timchalk and Nolan, (1997); [c]Carmichael et al. (1989)
[d]Renal clearance adjusted for body weight.

Table 2. Selected comparative species 2,4-D pharmacokinetic parameters calculated from the literature.

Parameters	Units	Mice[a]	Mice[b]	Rats[c]
Body weight (Bdwt)	Kg	0.02	0.02	0.2
Dose	mg kg^{-1}	1	5	5
Renal clearance (Clr)	mL hr^{-1}	1.56	1.29	7.48
Renal clearance (Clr)[g]	mL hr^{-1} kg^{-1}	78	64.5	37.4
Volume distribution (Vd)	L	0.002	0.003	0.02
Plasma half-life ($t_{1/2}$)	Hr	0.75	1.3	1.3

Parameters	Units	Dogs[d]	Pigs[e]	Calves[e]	Humans[f]
Body weight (Bdwt)	Kg	11	23	60	80
Dose	mg kg^{-1}	1	50	50	5
Renal clearance (Clr)	mL hr^{-1}	10.47	483	1506	1384
Renal clearance (Clr)[g]	mL hr^{-1} kg^{-1}	0.95	21	25.1	17.3
Volume distribution (Vd)	L	1.22	4.6	10.9	21.2
Plasma half-life ($t_{1/2}$)	Hr	31	6.6	5	11.6

[a]Grizzle *et al.* (1996); [b]Eiseman, (1984); [c]Kim *et al.* (1994); [d]Timchalk (1994); [e]Erne (1966); [f]Sauerhoff *et al.* (1977). [g] Renal clearance adjusted for body weight.

monkey and human with dogs having the longest half-life (25 hr). Likewise the 2,4-D $t_{1/2}$ for plasma elimination ranged from 0.75 to 11.6 hr in mice, rats, pigs, calves and humans and generally increased as a function of body weight. The dog was a particularly interesting exception with a 2,4-D plasma $t_{1/2}$ of 31 hr. These data were also compared utilizing allometric equations to appropriately scale between species based on their body weight to provide a more meaningful evaluation of the comparative species pharmacokinetics.

Inter-species pharmacokinetic scaling. Despite clear differences in appearance, mammals have similar physiology, biochemical and cellular structures and functions (Mordenti, 1986). Species comparison of the parameters obtained on compartmental analysis requires appropriate scaling in order to be meaningful. To adequately compare the underlying pharmacokinetic similarities and differences between species, the pharmacokinetic parameters

Table 3. Allometric equations for pharmacokinetic parameters: $Y = \alpha W^{\beta}$.

	Triclopyr[a]		2,4-D		ACPA[b]	
Parameter (Y)	α	β	α	β	α	β
Volume distribution (Vd)[c]	0.08	0.74	0.12	1.11	0.74	0.98
Renal Clearance (Clr)[d]	86	3.44[e]	37.4	0.86	3.44[e]	0.80[e]
Half-life ($t_{1/2}$)[d]	4.68	2.81	2.14	0.27	2.81	0.16

[a] Timchalk and Nolan (1997); [b] Cherkofsky (1995); [c]Included all species; [d]Excluding dog; [e]Calculated as plasma clearance.

must be appropriately scaled utilizing an allometric approach (Boxenbaum, 1982; Mordenti, 1986). Inter-species scaling has been extensively utilized to compare the pharmacokinetics and metabolism of pharmaceutical agents (Boxenbaum, 1982). In addition, these scaling approaches are being incorporated into risk assessment procedures to more accurately extrapolate dosimetry across species (Rees and Hattis, 1994). The allometric equation describing the relationship between body weight (W, in kg) and variable parameter Y is described in eq. 1. The allometric coefficient and allometric exponent are represented by α as the y-intercept and β as the slope, respectively.

$$Y=\alpha W^{\beta} \quad (1)$$

For the triclopyr and 2,4-D pharmacokinetic analysis, the variable parameter Y (Vd ,Clr, or $t_{1/2}$) was fit to eq. 1 by log-linear least square regression analysis. For each variable parameter a determination was made on whether to include the dog data in the analysis based on the goodness of fit.

A species comparison of the Vd, Cl_r, and $t_{1/2}$ versus body weight for triclopyr and 2,4-D is presented in Figure 2 and 3 and the allometric equations are presented in Table 3. The volume of distribution for triclopyr (Figure 2A) was well described for all species by the equation $Vd= 0.08W^{1.22}$. The relationship between renal clearance (mL h^{-1}) and body weight for rat, monkey and human was well described by the equation $Cl_r=86W^{0.78}$ (Figure 2B). The renal clearance of triclopyr in the dog, was clearly lower than in rat, monkey or human and was not adequately described like the other species by scaling to body weight. Likewise, analysis of elimination half-life versus body weight (Figure 2C) also indicated the dog was an outlier; if the dog was excluded, the relationship for the other species was described by the equation $t_{1/2}= 4.68W^{0.06}$.

The Vd for 2,4-D was relatively small and was well described for all species by the equation $Vd = 0.12\ W^{1.11}$ (Figure 3A). The relationship between renal Clr (mL hr^{-1}) and body weight for mice, rats, pigs, calves and humans was well described by the equation $Clr = 37\ W^{0.86}$ (Figure 3B). The Clr of 2,4-D in the dog was clearly lower than in all other species and was not adequately described by scaling. Likewise, analysis of elimination $t_{1/2}$ versus body weight (Figure 3C) also indicated that the dog was an outlier; if the dog was excluded, the relationship for the other species was well described by the equation $t_{1/2}=2.14\ W^{0.27}$.

It is proposed that the greater sensitivity of the dog to renal functional changes are primarily due to the dog's low capacity, relative to other species (including humans), to excrete organic acids. This hypothesis suggests that the comparative species response observed with triclopyr and 2,4-D should

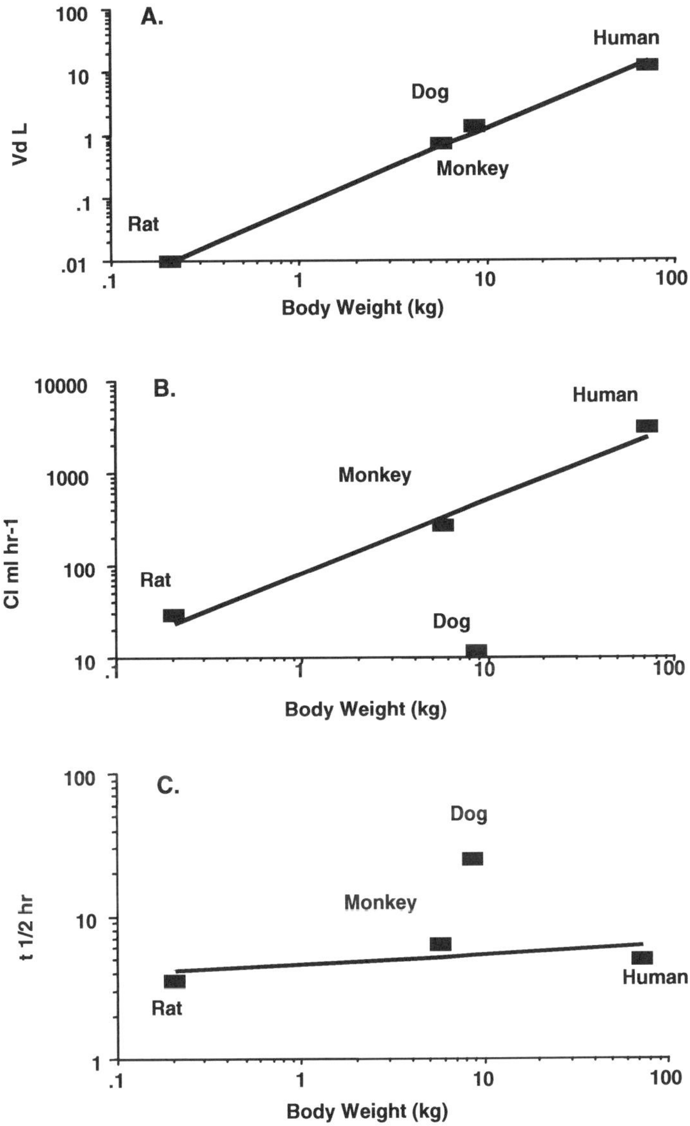

Figure 2. Triclopyr allometric relationship between body weight and (A) volume of distribution Vd (all species); (B) renal clearance Clr (excluding dog); and (C) elimination half-life t1/2 (excluding dog). This figure was adapted with permission from Timchalk and Nolan (1997).

also be seen with other organic acids. In this regard, the organic acid 1-aminocyclopropanecarboxylic acid (ACPA) which is a partial neurochemical receptor agonist having neuroprotective, antidepressant, and anxiolytic efficacy has undergone a similar allometric analysis (Cherkofsky, 1995). An inter-species allometric pharmacokinetic comparison of ACPA in mice, rats, monkeys, dogs and humans produced results strikingly similar to those obtained with 2,4-D, and triclopyr (*ibid*).

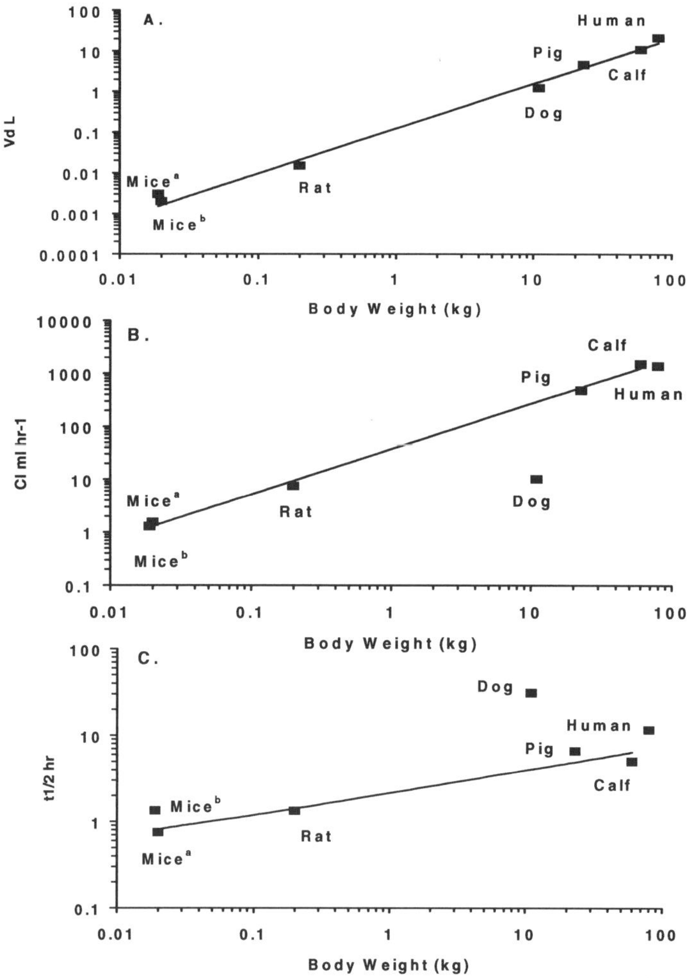

Figure 3. 2,4-D allometric relationship between body weight and (A) volume of distribution Vd (all species); (B) renal clearance Clr (excluding dog); and (C) elimination half-life t1/2 (excluding dog).

This comparison of selected allometrically scaled pharmacokinetic parameters highlights the observed species differences in the renal elimination of triclopyr, 2,4-D and the organic acid ACPA. This comparison was done with the low doses since comparisons at dose levels where the pharmacokinetics are nonlinear must be qualified by the dose. The allometric equations for Vd, Clr, and $t_{1/2}$ for triclopyr and 2,4-D are similar to reported exponents for other organic acids (see Table 3) (Timchalk and Nolan, 1997; Cherkofsky, 1995; Mordenti, 1986; Boxenbaum, 1982).

The good correlation for Vd across species is consistent with results seen with all three organic acids (Timchalk and Nolan, 1997; Cherkofsky, 1995). For each of the organic acids, the allometric exponents (β) for the Vd was close to unity (i.e.1.0) ranging from 0.95 to 1.11. This supports the conclusion that the Vd for each of the chemicals is proportional to body weight (Cherkofsky, 1995). In all species, the Vd was relatively small and equivalent to the volume of the blood and extracellular water as previously noted for triclopyr and 2,4-D in humans (Sauerhoff *et al.*, 1977; Carmichael *et al.*, 1988; Gehring *et al.*, 1973). In contrast, the allometric relationship between Clr and $t_{1/2}$ corroborated that the dog has a low capacity to eliminate organic acids like 2,4-D, triclopyr, and ACPA. The allometric coefficients (α) describing the y-intercept varies for each chemical; whereas, the allometric exponents (β) describing the slopes of the lines are comparable across species for a given parameter. For example, the allometric exponents (β) for Clr ranged from 0.63 - 0.86 which is consistent with the range of 0.66 - 0.92 that was reported in the literature for the clearance of other chemicals (Cherkofsky, 1995). Likewise, the exponents for $t_{1/2}$ ranged from 0.06 - 0.27 which was comparable to the 0.06 - 0.43 that was also previously reported (*ibid.*). This consistency of the allometric relationships between these organic acids supports the relevance of utilizing allometric scaling to compare pharmacokinetic parameters across species.

These comparative pharmacokinetics and allometric scaling results provide strong support for the position that in the dog the pharmacokinctics of triclopyr and 2,4-D are uniquely different than other species, including humans.

5.5 How are organic acids cleared in the kidney of dogs and excreted in the urine?

The renal handling of both endogenous and exogenous (drugs and chemicals) organic acids has been extensively studied in numerous species including the dog (Foreman, 1984; Rowland and Tozer 1996; Weiner, 1973). The appearance of an organic acid in the urine is the net result of glomerular filtration, tubular secretion and re-absorption (Rowland and Towzer, 1996).

For organic acids, like triclopyr and 2,4-D, that are eliminated primarily unmetabolized in the urine, at low dose levels the rate of urinary excretion is directly proportional to their plasma concentration. A reduction in the renal clearance of an organic acid will result in higher blood concentrations and slower elimination from the body. This is consistent with the observed nonlinear pharmacokinetics with increasing doses of these organic acids. To provide some understand of the clearance mechanism for these organic acids, renal clearance studies were conducted in the dog with triclopyr (Timchalk, *et al.*, 1997).

Glomerular filtration is a process in which the plasma entering the glomerulus is passively filtered producing a filtrate that has a composition comparable to plasma, but contains little if any protein. Therefore, only chemicals and drugs that are free i.e. not bound to plasma proteins, are cleared by glomerular filtration. It has been shown in numerous species including rats, goats, dogs, and humans that organic acids like 2,4-D and triclopyr are extensively bound (90 – 99%) to plasma proteins (Hook *et al.*, 1976; Braunlich *et al.*, 1989; Orberg, 1980; Piper *et al.*, 1973; Timchalk and Nolan, 1997). To further illustrate this point the extent of triclopyr plasma protein binding, in the dog, as a function of the blood concentration is depicted in Figure 4. Over the concentrations evaluated, the amount of unbound triclopyr (free) in the plasma ranged from a high of only 7% to a low

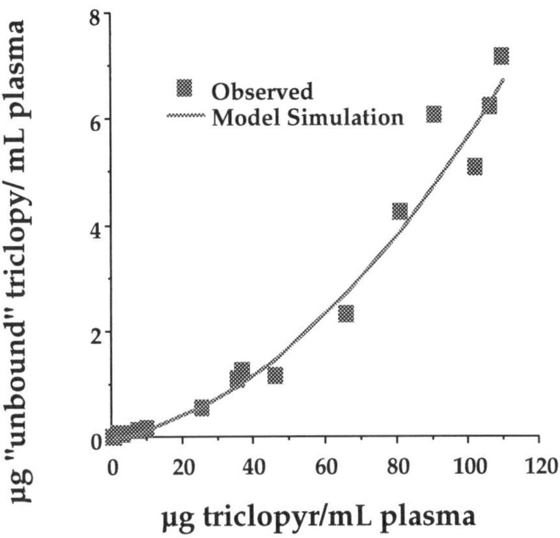

Figure 4. Observed and best fit plasma protein binding of triclopyr as a function of the plasma triclopyr concentration. This figure was adapted with permission from Timchalk and Nolan (1997).

of 0.88% (Timchalk and Nolan, 1997). Since only the "free" chemical (not bound to plasma protein) is available for passive filtration it has been suggested that filtration represents a relatively minor component of the overall renal clearance mechanism for organic acid herbicides (Gehring and Betso, 1978; Piper *et al.*, 1973; Hook *et al.* 1974, Orberg, 1980; Timchalk and Nolan, 1997).

On the other hand, active renal tubular secretion is of particular importance for plasma clearance of organic acids (Renwick, 1994). Secretion occurs in the proximal tubules and is an active saturable process involving carrier proteins having broad substrate affinities. Although organic acids, like triclopyr and 2,4-D are extensively but reversibly bound to plasma proteins they are readily dissociated from the proteins, transported across the proximal tubule epithelium and secreted into the tubule lumen (Weiner, 1973). The renal organic acid secretory system is believed to be the primary mechanism for the plasma clearance and elimination of phenoxy- and pyridinyloxyacetic acids (Erne, 1966; Gehring and Betso, 1978; Piper *et al.*, 1973; Hook *et al.*, 1976; Orberg, 1980; Timchalk and Nolan, 1997). *In vitro* renal cortical slice and isolated renal tubule systems have been used to facilitate the understanding of the renal tubule secretory mechanism of 2,4-D and related organic acids in the rat, dog, rabbit and winter flounder (Dawson and Renfro, 1993; Baaunlick *et al.* 1989; Hook *et al.*, 1974; Brendt and Koschier, 1973). 2,4-D demonstrates non-linear pharmacokinetics and this dose-dependent decreased clearance is proposed to be due to a limited capacity to actively secrete the acid at high plasma concentrations (Gehring and Betso, 1978). Likewise, it has been demonstrated that the renal uptake and clearance of 2,4-D and triclopyr by the organic acid secretory system can be competitively inhibited by other organic acids (e.g. p-aminohippuric acid (PAH), PSP and probenecid) (Koschier and Berndt, 1977; Piper *et al.*, 1973; Hook *et al.*, 1976; Berndt and Koschier, 1973; Koschier *et al.*, 1978; Timchalk *et al.*, 1997).

Once the organic acid is within the tubule lumen both active and passive processes are available to facilitate reabsorption (Rowlen and Tozer, 1996; Foreman, 1984). This bi-directional transport has been demonstrated in numerous species for a number of organic acids including: triclopyr, citrate, lactate, α-ketoglutarate and ketone bodies, PAH, salicylate and a number of differing classes of antibiotics and diuretics (Weiner, 1973; Foreman, 1984; Timchalk and Nolan, 1997). The extent of reabsorption is dependent upon a number of factors such as, degree of ionization, concentration, molecular weight, urine flow and pH (Rowlen and Tozer, 1996). Hook *et al.* (1976) reported that the renal clearance of 2,4,5-trichlorophenxoyacetic acids was extremely slow in the dog and suggested that passive reabsorption of the herbicide contributed to the slow clearance. This position was further supported by the observation that by increasing the pH of the urine, the organic acid clearance was increased. A recent study with triclopyr also suggests that tubular reabsorption occurs, but was evident primarily at high plasma triclopyr concentrations in the dog (Timchalk and Nolan, 1997). These data support the involvement of bi-directional transport of organic acids in the renal tubules of the dog.

The excretion of organic acids like triclopyr and 2,4-D in the urine is the net result of filtration, secretion and reabsorption processes. To help exemplify this point, the ratio of renal clearance/glomerular filtration (Clr/Clf) for triclopyr versus the plasma concentration is plotted in Figure 5 (Timchalk and Nolan, 1997). This ratio illustrates the net direction (secretion or reabsorption) of renal transport. When reabsorption exceeds secretion, the renal clearance will be less than glomerular filtration. On the other hand, a value greater than one indicates net secretion. Renal clearance is influenced by numerous factors including, dose, dose-rate, extent of plasma protein-binding, affinity and capacity of the tubular secretory system for the acid, urinary flow and urinary pH. Although renal clearance mechanisms for organic acids are ubiquitous in mammalian species there appears to be clear qualitative discrepancies between species that may account for observed differences in clearance.

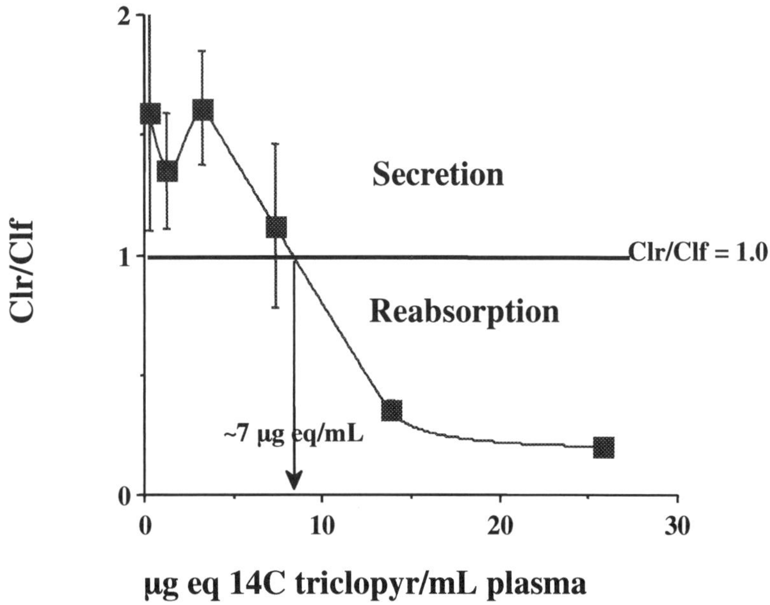

Figure 5. Average triclopyr clearance ratio curves obtained from male Beagle dogs. This figure was adapted with permission from Timchalk and Nolan (1997).

In the case of triclopyr, we have proposed a functional model (see Figure 6) to describe the renal elimination of this organic acid; it is similar to a model used to describe the transport of urate in dogs (Foreman, 1984). Based on comparable modes of action it is reasonable to assume that qualitatively other organic acids, such as 2,4-D, will be cleared similarly. At low plasma concentrations (Figure 6B), the organic acid is cleared by active secretion and filtration with secretion accounting for a relatively larger percentage of the overall clearance. With increasing plasma concentrations (Figure 6C) active secretion becomes saturated, hence a greater percentage of the clearance is associated with filtration. At very high plasma concentrations (Figure 6D) an even greater percentage of the organic acid would be filtered while the active secretion remains saturated. The increased concentration of the acid within the tubular lumen would also create a greater diffusion gradient resulting in a significant re-absorption of the organic acid.

A number of *in vivo* organic acid clearance studies provide critical insight into the mechanisms for the renal clearance of organic acids in the dog. The results seen with triclopyr are consistent with other observations in dogs with a variety of organic acids including: citrate, lactate, PAH, PSP, and iodopyracet (Weiner, 1973; Foreman, 1984). For example, iodopyracet and PAH are both actively secreted by low-capacity high-affinity renal transport systems, similar to triclopyr. Likewise, urate, ascorbic acid and salicylates clearly demonstrate bi-directional transport. These studies all support a renal clearance mechanism for organic acids in the dog that entails glomerular filtration of the non-plasma-bound fraction, a saturable active transport process and reabsorption within the renal tubules.

5.6 Are renal functional changes a toxicological response or a physiological adaptation associated with the excretion of organic acids?

In dogs administered triclopyr at doses that do not result in any pathology, slight functional changes were observed and included a reduction in PSP excretion and a slight increase in urinary BUN and creatinine (1988; unpublished report of The Dow Chemical Co., Midland, MI). The question this data raises is whether the observed changes in PSP, BUN and creatinine are representative of a toxicological response or a physiological adaptation? To address this question comparative renal function studies were conducted in both dogs and monkeys following repeated administration (up to 100 days) of triclopyr at doses ranging from 5 – 20 mg/kg/day (Timchalk *et al.*, 1997).

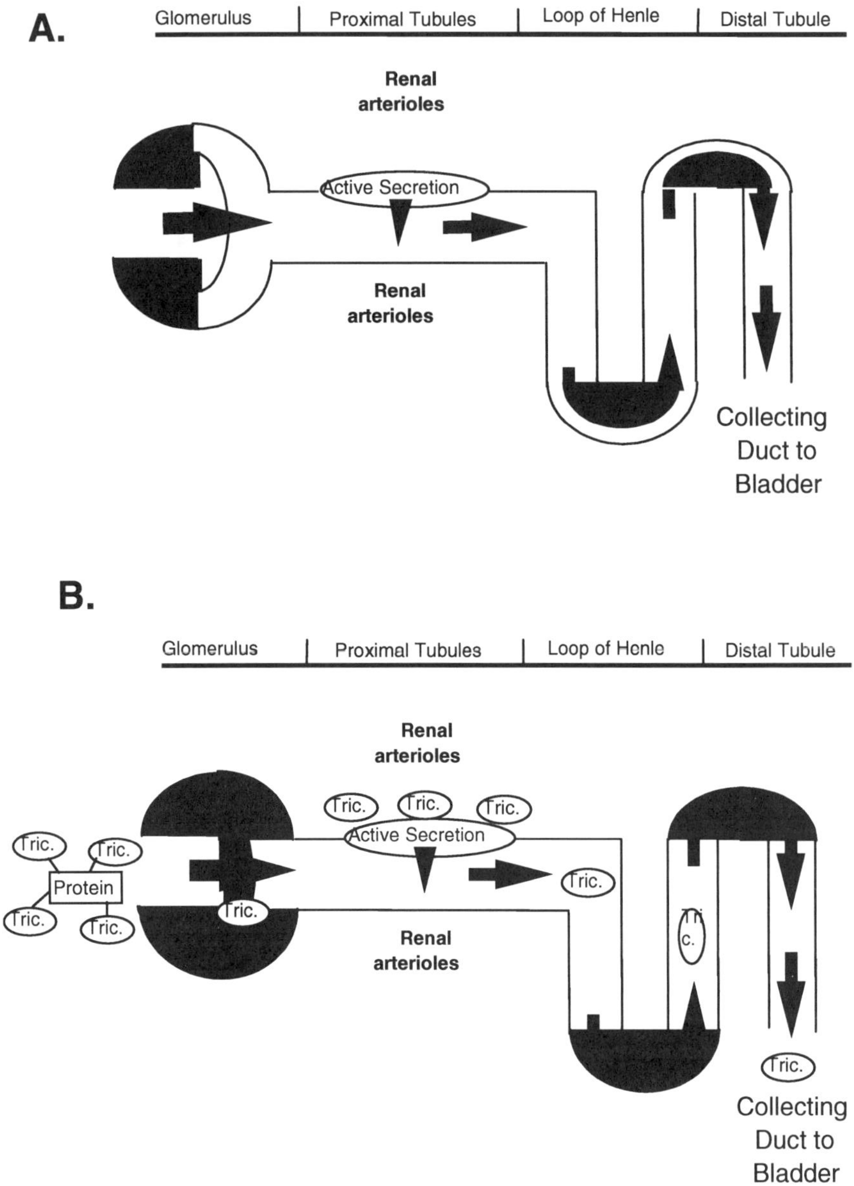
A.
Glomerulus
Proximal Tubules
Loop of Henle
Distal Tubule
Renal arterioles
Active Secretion
Renal arterioles
Collecting Duct to Bladder
B.
Glomerulus
Proximal Tubules
Loop of Henle
Distal Tubule
Renal arterioles
Tric.
Tric.
Tric.
Active Secretion
Tric.
Tric.
Protein
Tric.
Tric.
Tric.
Tric.
Renal arterioles
Tri c.
Tric.
Collecting Duct to Bladder

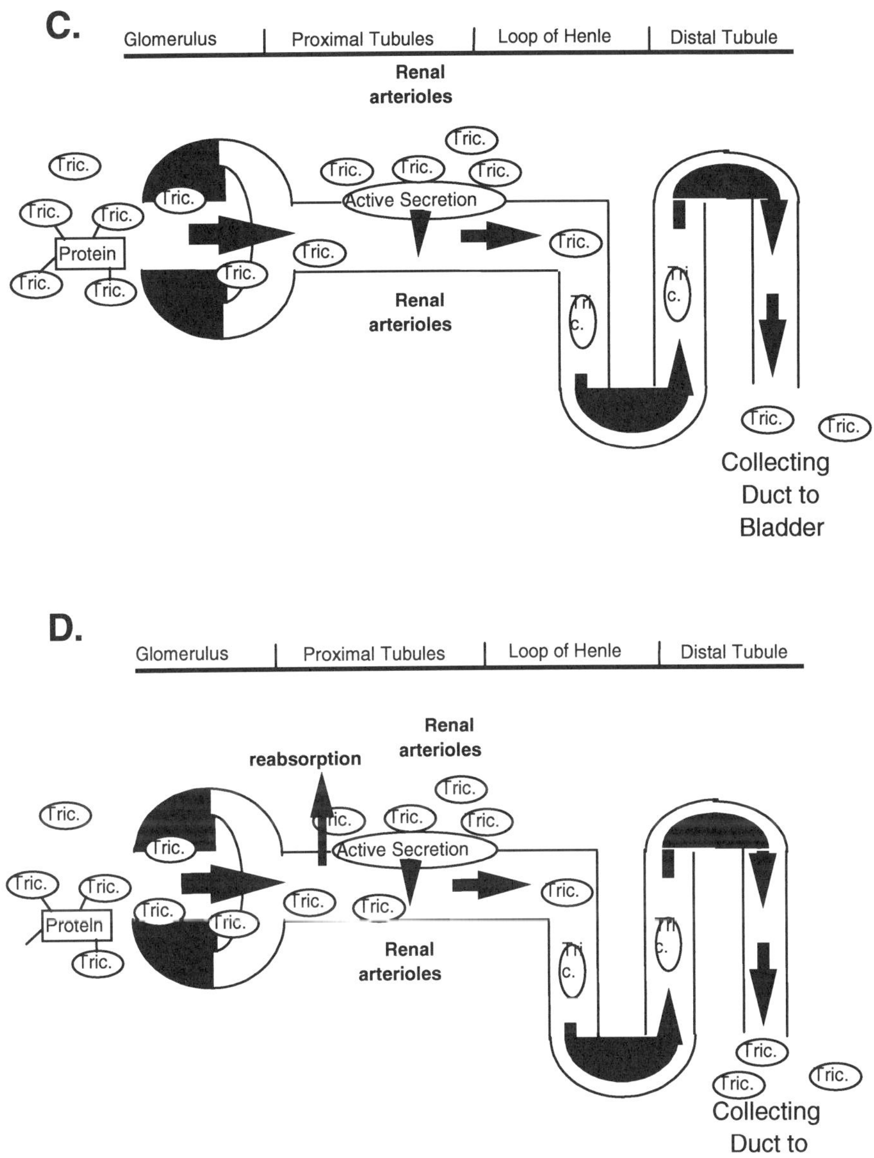

Figure 6. Proposed model for the renal handling of triclopyr in the dog. (A) kidney nephron, (B) low concentration, (C) intermediate concentration, and (D) high concentration. This figure was adapted with permission from Timchalk and Nolan (1997).

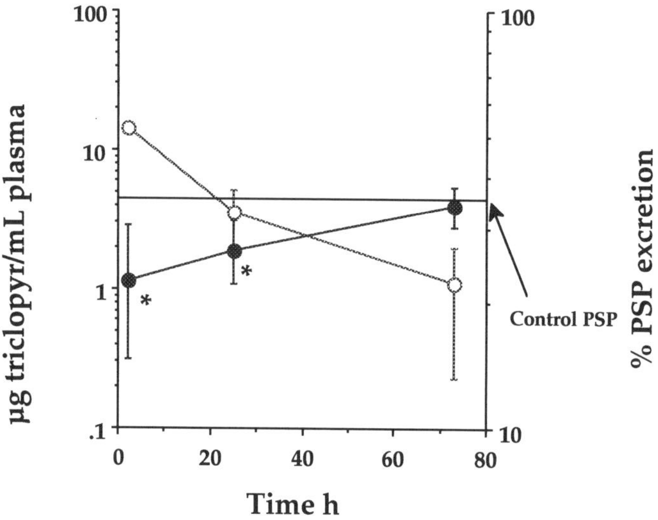

Figure 7. Relationship between plasma triclopyr concentration (O) and percent PSP excretion (•) in Beagle dogs administered a single oral dose of 5 mg triclopyr/kg of body weight. The average control percentage of PSP excretion was 36 ± 5%. Values identified as statistically significant are identified with an asterisk (*). This figure was adapted with permission from Timchalk et al.(1997).

In monkeys triclopyr did not produce a decrease in PSP excretion. However in dogs, PSP excretion was decreased and inversely related to the plasma triclopyr concentration (see Figure 7). These results are consistent with numerous studies that demonstrated a decreased renal clearance of organic acids, including PSP, when co-administered with other organic acids (Russel, *et al.*, 1989; Mann *et al.*, 1991; Foreman, 1984; Weiner, 1973). This effect of an organic acid on PSP excretion is consistent with a physiological response due to competition of triclopyr and PSP for the same active secretory site. In addition, monkeys appear to be insensitive to the effects of triclopyr on the active secretory process even at doses fourfold higher than the effective dose in the dog (Timchalk *et al.*, 1997).

Both BUN and serum creatinine are routinely utilized to evaluate renal function although these parameters have limited sensitivity since renal function must be decreased to 25% of normal or less to be detected by these measurements (Finco, 1989; Shuster and Seldin, 1992). As can be seen in Figures 8 and 9 repeated administration of triclopyr to both dogs and monkeys had no biologically meaningful impact on either creatinine or BUN (Timchalk *et al.*, 1997). The values obtained in both species were well within their normal range (Osborne *et al.*, 1972; Duncan and Prasse, 1986). These results in both dogs and monkeys at doses as high as 20 mg/kg/day

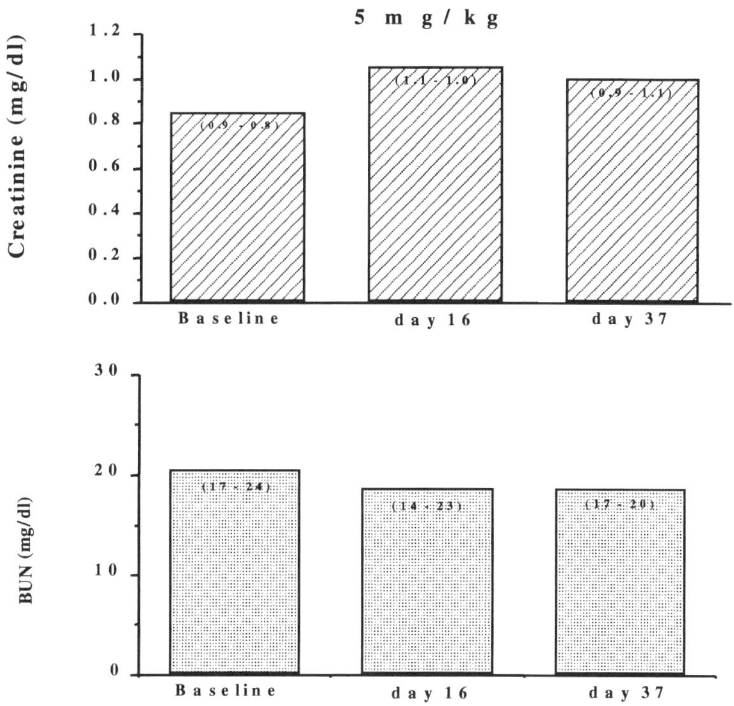

Figure 8. Endogenous creatinine (A) and BUN (B) concentrations in male Beagle dogs administered triclopyr at a dose of 5 mg/kg/day in their diet for 47 days. The values represent mean for two animals and individual animal data are presented in parentheses. This figure was adapted with permission from Timchalk et al.(1997).

suggest that repeated exposure to triclopyr had no effect on normal kidney function in either species. Kidney toxicity related changes in serum creatinine and BUN are only observed in the presence of significant renal damage (i.e. 70% or greater of the nephrons are damaged). Therefore, the most reasonable explanation for the slight changes in BUN and creatinine levels in the chronic dog study is that they primarily represent a physiological adaptation and not toxicity.

5.7 What potential mechanism(s) may be responsible for the reduced elimination of organic acids in the dog?

It has previously been shown that the excretion of organic acids in the urine is the net result of filtration, secretion and reabsorption processes. It is proposed that the mechanism of organic acid excretion in the dog is similar to those utilized by other species. However, quantitative differences exist which limits the dogs capacity to excrete organic acids relative to other species. Hook *et al.* (1974) compared the *in vitro* transport of the organic acid 2,4,5-T in rat and dog renal cortex in an attempt to provide perspective on the species differences in biological $t_{1/2}$. They reported that rat and dog renal cortical slices both actively accumulated 2,4,5-T.

However, in rat tissue the peak slice/medium (S/M) ratio was ~14, whereas in dog kidney slices the highest ratio obtained was ~8.6. These results indicate that the dog has a lower capacity to actively excrete this organic acid relative to the rat. It is reasonable to infer that a similar response would be seen with other organic acids like triclopyr or 2,4-D. It is also reasonable to anticipate that filtration and reabsorption processes may contribute to the lower elimination in the dog. The Clr of the organic acid ACPA

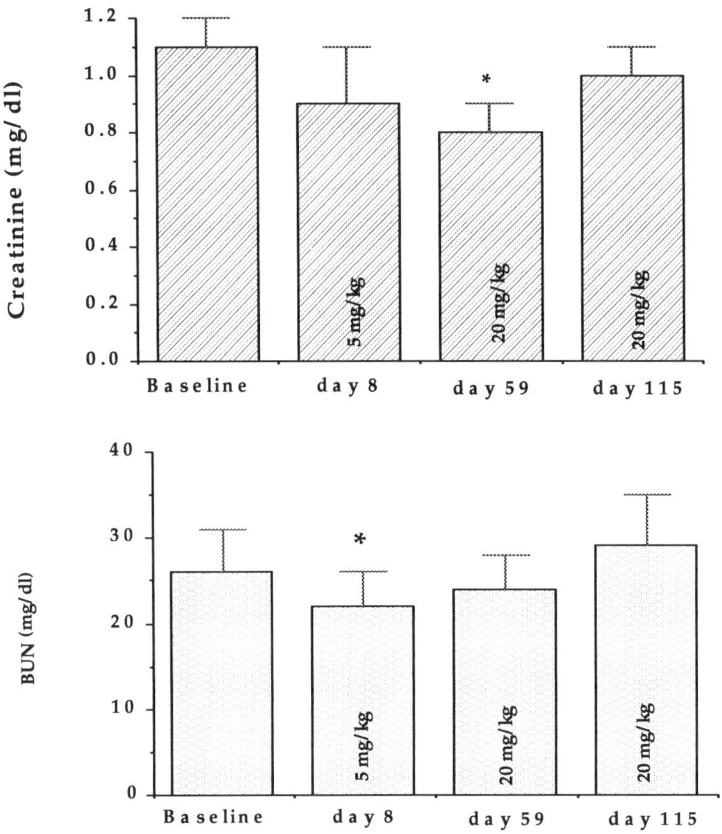

Figure 9. Endogenous creatinine (A) and BUN (B) concentrations in male Rhesus monkeys repeatedly administered triclopyr at doses of 5 mg/kg/day for 28 days followed by an additional 102 days at 20 mg/kg/day. Values represent mean ± SD for four animals. Values identified as statistically significant are identified with an asterisk (*). This figure was adapted with permission from Timchalk et al.(1997).

was only 16% of the glomerular filtration rate (GFR) in the dog; whereas, in the rat the clearance was ~63% of the GFR (Cherkofsky, 1995). It was proposed that this low Clr in the dog was due to reabsorption in the proximal tubules resulting in a slower Clr and longer $t_{1/2}$. Timchalk and Nolan (1997) conducted an *in vivo* renal Clr study with the organic acid triclopyr in dogs. They reported a dose-dependent non-linear decrease in plasma protein-binding and significant increases in tubular reabsorption of triclopyr at higher doses, which appears to account for the observed pharmacokinetics.

Based on the current understanding of the mode of renal clearance for related phenoxyacetic acid herbicides and other organic acids, it is reasonable to infer that triclopyr and 2,4-D are handled by mammals in a similar fashion. The most likely mechanism responsible for the unique sensitivity of the dog, is a low capacity to actively secrete the organic acid from the kidney.

5.8 Is the dog toxicity data obtained with either triclopyr or 2,4-D of any relevance for the extrapolation of human health risk?

This comparative species evaluation of the pharmacokinetics and renal elimination of the pyridinyloxy- and phenoxyacetic acid herbicides triclopyr and 2,4-D questions the relevance of using dog toxicity data for the extrapolation of human health risk. The dog is unique because of its limited capacity to excrete organic acids relative to other species. The steady-state body burden for the organic acids are inversely proportional to the capacity of an organism to excrete them. Therefore, the dog is an inappropriate model for human risk assessment since it will have exceedingly higher body burdens of these organic acids due to its limited clearance capacity. Humans not only eliminate triclopyr and 2,4-D much faster than the dog, but exposure from occupational and home and garden use is low (Munro *et al.*, 1992; Middendorf *et al.*, 1994), so that its elimination is clearly within the linear kinetic range.

To provide additional perspective the allometric equation describing triclopyr and 2,4-D renal Clr were used to project their Clr in dogs assuming they had a similar capacity as other species to clear organic acids (see Figure 10). The results suggest that for the dog to be of any relevance (from a pharmacokinetic perspective) for extrapolation to humans, a 38 (12 vs. 450 ml hr^{-1}) and 30 fold greater renal Clr capacity is needed (10.5 vs. ~300 ml hr^{-1}) for triclopyr and 2,4-D, respectively. Based on these pharmacokinetic comparisons it appears obvious that the toxicity data for animals such as rats or mice having a similar rate of Clr scaled by body weight would be a significantly more relevant than the dog as a starting point for extrapolation of human health risk from triclopyr and 2,4-D.

The current risk assessment paradigm for non-cancer endpoints generally assumes a threshold of response, and therefore utilizes a safety factor approach for establishing exposure guidelines (Rees and Hattis, 1994). The methodology involves the concept of a reference dose (RfD) which is defined as an estimate of a daily exposure to the human population which is without appreciable risk during a life-time (Rees and Hattis, 1994; EPA, 1989). The RfD is calculated by dividing a NOEL dose obtained from an "appropriate" animal study by a calculated uncertainty factor. The magnitude of the safety factor (~10 – 1000 fold) is determined by a number of parameters including, the ability to extrapolate from animal to human, the variability in human sensitivity and the adequacy of available toxicological databases on the chemical of interest (Rees and Hattis, 1994; Derelanko, 1995). The RfD approach is critically dependent upon the NOEL that is chosen (Rees and Hattis, 1994), including the relevance of specific animal species for human risk extrapolation. The implications are particularly relevant for triclopyr, 2,4-D and related organic acids where the lowest NOELs are obtained in dogs and appear to correlate well with their slower clearance of organic acids. The lack of a pharmacokinetic concordance between the dog and other mammals calls into question the relevance of utilizing the dog for evaluation of human health risk from exposure to these organic acids. Therefore, from a risk assessment perspective, it would seem prudent to utilize toxicity data from other species (e.g. rodents) for establishing NOELs for RfD determinations. However, if the dog NOEL is utilized for establishing an RfD the need for an additional uncertainty factor for animal to human pharmacokinetic differences is not warranted, since, from a pharmacokinetic perspective, the dog is clearly more sensitive than humans. Finally, interspecies pharmacokinetic comparisons of those mammalian species utilized for toxicological testing may provide critically important perspective on the relevance of specific species for human health risk assessment and help facilitate choosing the most appropriate animal species for establishing a NOEL for the RfD.

5.9 Regulatory Outcomes

Triclopyr. The U.S. Environmental Protection Agency (EPA) reduced the RfD for triclopyr in 1994 from 0.025 to 0.005 mg/kg/day based on a NOEL in the dog chronic toxicity study of 0.5 mg/kg/day and an uncertainty factor of 100 to account for both inter-species extrapolation and intra-species variability. Increases in serum creatinine and blood urea nitrogen (BUN) were observed at the next higher dose level of 2.5 mg/kg/day.

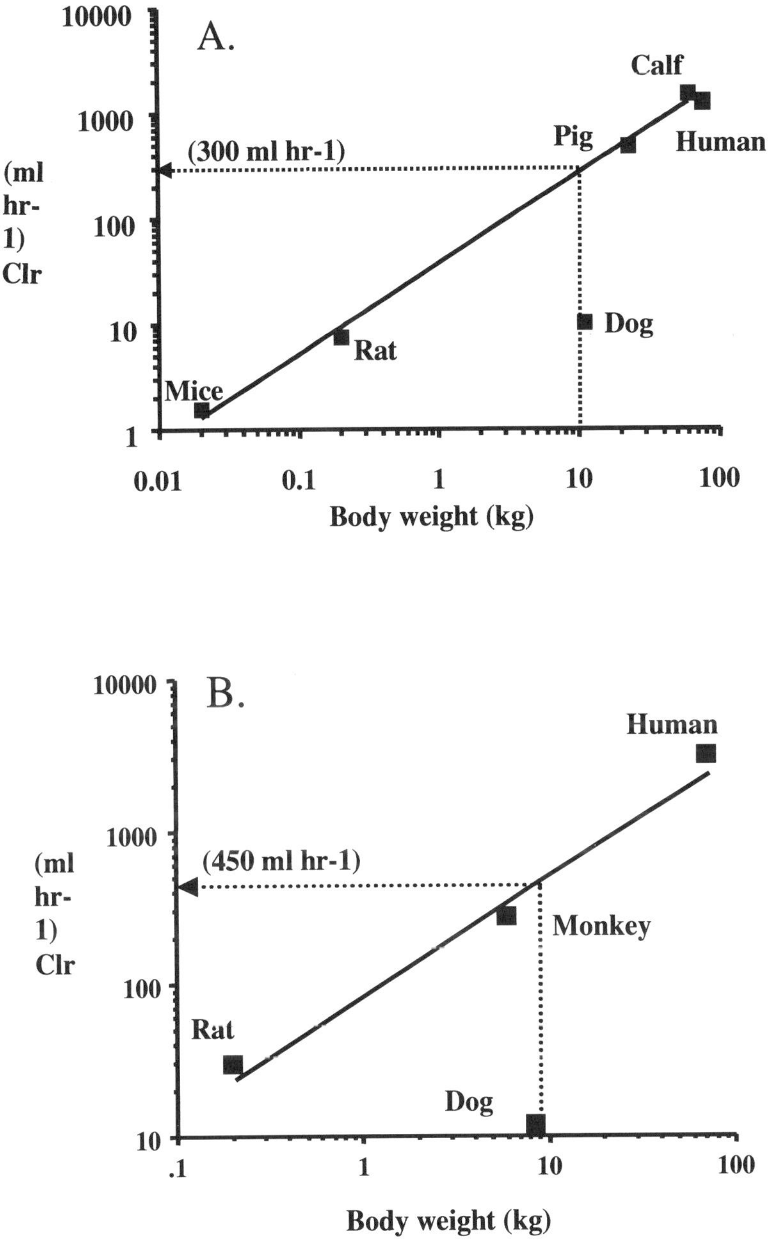

Figure 10. Projected renal clearance (Clr) of 2,4-D (A) and triclopyr (B) in the dog assuming Clr was scaled to body weight in the dog.

Dow AgroSciences petitioned the Agency in 1996 to reconsider the RfD for triclopyr based on the position that the increases in creatinine and BUN in the dog at 2.5 mg/kg/day were within the biological range of variation for these parameters in dogs (based on historical control data) and were not evidence of kidney toxicity. The company supported their position on the basis that changes in serum creatinine and BUN would only be expected in the presence of significant renal damage (i.e., 70% or greater of nephrons are damaged) and, in fact, there was no evidence of kidney pathology on the chronic dog study. Furthermore, a test of urine concentrating ability in a 228-day toxicity study in dogs did not detect any decrement in the ability of the kidneys to concentrate urine.

Dow AgroSciences also submitted the studies described in the current publication to the Agency in support of the argument that the dog is an inappropriate model based on the limited capacity of this species to excrete organic acids. After comprehensive reevaluation of all the toxicological data, the EPA concluded that:

1. The biological/toxicological significance of the kidney effects in the chronic dog study is questionable and they appear to be the result of physiological adaptation and may not be of toxicological significance.
2. The dog is not the appropriate animal model for kidney toxicity testing of triclopyr.
3. The RfD for triclopyr should be 0.05 mg/kg/day based on a reproductive toxicity study in rats with a NOEL of 5 mg/kg/day and an uncertainty factor of 100. The kidneys of P1 and P2 adult rats on this study had mild degeneration of the proximal tubules at the next higher dose level of 25 mg/kg/day.

The additional triclopyr data and mechanistic perspective provided to the EPA, with emphasis on comparative species pharmacokinetics, provided the basis for the EPA's decision to revise the RfD for triclopyr from 0.005 mg/kg/day based on the chronic dog study to 0.05 mg/kg/day based on the adults in the rat reproduction study. The increase in the RfD provides an additional 10X margin of safety in many risk assessments and environmental impact statements for triclopyr.

2,4-D. The first 2,4-D European Union (EU) dossier was submitted to the regulatory authorities with an Allowable Occupational Exposure Limit (AOEL) that was derived from the results of a chronic study conducting in the rat. In this initial dossier the dog species was not included based on its low capacity to excrete organic acids. This conclusion was supported by data that compared the 2,4-D pharmacokinetic pattern in the rat, dog and man with 2,4,5-T data as well as other relevant literature. However, this submission did not take advantage of the allometric scaling approaches that are presented in this paper. Overall, these arguments were not convincing to the regulatory authority in Greece, who was the primary rapporter member state (RMS) responsible for 2,4-D. Consequently the proposed AOEL was not accepted and a new one was set using both the dog and the rodent sub-chronic studies. Using this new AOEL, the operator exposures were not acceptable under any potential use scenario. Therefore, in order to maintain 2,4-D registration, data was needed to support increasing the AOEL and/or decreasing the dermal penetration factor used in the risk assessment. The strategy entailed working on three relevant issues simultaneously:

1. Provide a more convincing argument on the non-relevance of the dog species for human risk assessment.
2. Provide a convincing argument to support a higher rodent sub-chronic NOEL.
3. Establish a lower dermal penetration factor that the default 10%.

To address the dog issue there was a need to develop a more compelling scientific argument built around the application of allometric scaling to demonstrate a lack of relevance for human health risk assessment, as outlined in this paper. Secondly, while working primarily with the RMS (Greece), the strategy also entailed meeting or discussing the approach with experts from key EU member states, to at least obtain a non-official position on this issue.

The RMS and the majority of the member state experts accepted the results of the allometric scaling and agreed with the position that the dog was not a relevant species for extrapolation of 2,4-D risk to humans. This resulted in the RMS changing its initial position, opting to not use the dog toxicity data for setting an AOEL, but rather based the AOEL on the rodent data.

5.10 Utility of Comparative Pharmacokinetics

In this manuscript we have attempted to demonstrate the utility of a simple straightforward pharmacokinctic approach to provide important scientific perspective on the relevance of specific animal toxicity data for human health risk assessment. The approach that was successfully utilized required a fairly comprehensive pharmacokinetic data-base in which kinetic studies were conducted in multiple species including humans. On the other hand the success of this approach may likewise suggest that comparative species pharmacokinetic studies should be considered as an important complement to ongoing multiple species toxicity testing. This may be particularly important during the development of new chemistries where there is little if any understanding of mammalian toxicity.

It should be noted that this approach did entail a number of significant challenges. The pharmacokinetic data-base that was utilized to make the allometric comparisons ranged from recent studies to some conducted over 34 years ago. Hence the quality, availability and appropriateness of the data to the questions at hand were an issue. Secondly, other than the studies that we specifically conducted, there were significant challenges in piecing together a cohesive story from a variety of unrelated projects. On the other hand the fact that a diverse data set could be utilized to make a compelling integrated argument suggests that our approach has strong scientific merit. Finally, the focus of our effort was on the impact of species differences in renal clearance that was based on our understanding of how organic acids are excreted. This approach represents a concrete example of the utility of comparative pharamcokinetics for identifying unique species differences in toxicological response.

5.11 Summary & Conclusions

The results of this review and analysis support the hypothesis that the unique sensitivity of the dog to triclopyr and 2,4-D can be traced to the decreased capacity of the dog to excrete organic acids. The most likely mechanism responsible for this sensitivity, is a low capacity in the dog to actively secrete organic acids in the kidney. The allometric analysis of pharmacokinetic parameters for a number of related organic acids suggest that the low responsiveness of the dog is not compound specific. It appears to be associated with organic acids that share common pharmacokinetic properties, such as (1) extensive but reversible plasma protein-binding, (2) weak acids that are highly ionized at physiological pH, (3) limited metabolism of the parent acid, and (4) urinary excretion primarily involving a saturable active secretion. The results of the inter-species allometric analysis for several related organic acids are extremely similar and suggest that the dog is not a reasonable animal model for extrapolation of risk to humans for these organic acids. Therefore, based on this scientific evidence it would seem reasonable to use the toxicity data generated in rodents for RfD calculations and extrapolation of human health risk for organic acids.

5.12 References

Arnold, E. K. and Beasley, V. R. (1989). The pharmacokinetics of chlorinated phenoxy acid herbicides: a literature review. *Vet. Hum. Toxicol.*, 31 (2), 121 – 125.

Berndt, W. O. and Koschier, F. (1973). *In vitro* uptake of 2,4-dichlorphenoxyacetic acid (2,4-D) and 2,4,5-trichlorophenoxyacetic acid (2,4,5-T) by renal cortical tissue of rabbits and rats. *Toxicol. Appl. Pharmacol.*, 26, 559 – 570.

Boxenbaum, H. (1982). Interspecies scaling, allometry, physiological time and the ground plan of pharmacokinetics. J. Pharmacokinetics and Biopharmaceutics, 10(2), 201 – 227.

Braunlich, H., Bernhardt, H., and Bernhardt, I. (1989). Renal handling of 2-methyll-4-chloropheoxyacetic acid (MCPA) in rats. *J. Appl. Toxicol.*, 9(4), 255 – 258.

Carmichael, N. G., Nolan, R. J., Perkins, J. M., Davies, R., and Warrington, S. J. (1989). Oral and dermal pharmacokinetics of triclopyr in human volunteers. *Human Toxicol.*, 8, 431 – 437.

Charles, J. M., Bond, D. M., Jefferies, T. K., Yano, B. L., Stott, W.T., Johnson, K. A., Cunny, H. C., Wilson, R. D. and Bus, J. S. (1996a) Chronic dietary toxicity/oncogenicity studies on 2,4-dichlorophenoxyacetic acid in rodents. *Fund. Appl. Pharmacol.*, 33, 166 – 172.

Charles, J. M., Dalgard, D. W., Cunny, H. C., Wilson, R. D. and Bus, J. S. (1996b). Comparative subchronic and chronic dietary toxicity studies on 2,4-dichlorophenxoyacetic acid, amine and ester in the dog. *Fund. Appl. Pharmacol.*, 29, 78 – 85.

Cherkofsky, S. C. (1995). 1-Aminocyclopropanecarboxylic acid: mouse to man interspecies pharmacokinetic comparisons and allometric relationships. *J. Pharm. Sci.,* 84(10), 1231 – 1235.

Dalgaard-Mikkelsen, S., and Poulsen, E. (1962). Toxicology of herbicides. *Pharmac. Rev.*, 14, 225 – 250.

Dawson, M. J. and Renfro, J. L. (1993). Interaction of structurally similar pesticides with organic anion transport by primary cultures of winter flounder renal proximal tubule. *J. Pharmacol. Exper. Therap.*, 226 (2), 673 – 677.

Derelanko, M. J. (1995). Risk assessment. In: *CRC Handbook of Toxicology*, Ed. M. J. Derelanko and M. A. Hollinger, CRC Press Inc., Boca Raton, Fl., pp. 278 – 280.

Duncan, J. R. and Prasse, K. W. (1986). *Veterinary Laboratory Medicine- Clinical Pathology,* 2nd ed., Iowa State Univ. Press, Ames IA.

Eiseman, J. L. (1984). The pharmacokinetic evaluation of ^{14}C-2,4-dichlorophenoxyacetic acid (2,4-D) in the mouse. Final Report, Industry Task Force on 2,4-D Research Data, Midland, MI.

Eisenbrandt, D. L., Landry, T. D., Firchau, H. M., Tsuda, S. and Quast, J. F. (1988). Dietary chronic toxicity and oncogenicity studies of triclopyr in rats and mice. Toxicologist, 8: 704.

Environmental Protection Agency (EPA) (1995). RfD/Peer Review Report of Triclopyr (3,5,6-Trichloro-2-pyridinyloxyacetic acid) and Triethylamine Salt and Butoxyethylester of Triclopyr. Office of Prevention, Pesticides and Toxic Substances.

EPA (1989). Interim methods for development of inhalation reference doses. EPA/600/8-88/006F.

Erne, K. (1966). Distribution and elimination of chlorinated phenoxyacetic acids in animals. *ACTA Vet Scand.*, 7, 240 – 256.

Erne, K., and Sperber, I. (1974). Renal tubular transfer of phenoxyacetic acids in the chicken. *Acta Pharmacol. Toxicol.*, 35, 233 – 241.

Finco, D. R. (1989). Kidney function. In: *Clinical Biochemistry of Domestic Animals* (J. J. Kaneko, Ed.), pp. 496 – 542. Academic Press, New York.

Foreman, J. W. (1984). Renal handling of urate and other organic acids. In Canine nephrology (K.C. Bovee, Ed.), pp. 135 – 151. Harwal Publishing Co.

Gehring, P. J., Kramer, C. G., Schwetz, B. A., Rose, J. Q. and Rowe, V. K. (1973). The fate of 2,4,5-trichlorophenoxyacetic acid (2,4,5-T) following oral administration to man. Toxicol. Appl. Pharmacol., 26, 352 – 361.

Gehring, P.J., and Betso, J. E. (1978). Phenoxy acids: effects and fate in mammals. In *Chlorinated phenoxy acids and their dioxins* (C. Ramel Ed.), Vol. 27, pp. 122 – 133. Ecol. Bull., Stockholm.

Gorzinski, S. J., Kociba, R. J., Campbell, R. A., Smith, F. A., Nolan, R. J., and Eisenbrandt, D. L. (1987). Acute, pharmacokinetic and subchronic toxicological studies of 2,4-dichlorophenoxyacetic acid. *Fund. Appl. Toxicol.,* 9, 423 – 435.

Griffin, R. J., Godfrey, V. B., Kim, Y.C., and Burka, L. T. (1997). Sex dependent differences in the disposition of 2,4-dichlorophenoxyacetic acid in Sprague-Dawley rats, $B_6C_3F_1$ mice and Syrian hamsters. *Drug Metab. Disposition,* 25(9), 1065 – 1071.

Grizzle, T. B., Buckley-Kedderis, L., Collins, B. J., Goehl, T. J., Handy, R. W. and Marsman, D. S. (1995). Toxicokinetics of 2,4-dichlorophenoxyacetic acid (2,4-D) in rats, mice and hamsters. *The Inter. Cong. Toxicol.* VII, 47-P-9.

Hook, J. B., Bailie, M. D., Johnson, J. T., and Gehring, P. J. (1974). *In vitro* analysis of transport of 2,4,5-trichlorophenoxyacetic acid by rat and dog kidney. *Fd. Cosmet. Toxicol.,* 12, 209 – 218.

Hook, J. B., Cardona, R., Osborn, J. L. and Bailie, M. D. (1976). The renal handling of 2,4,5-trichlorophenoxyacetic acid (2,4,5-T) in the dog. Fd. Cosmet. Toxicol., 14, 19 – 23.

Kim, C. S., Gargas, M. L. and Andersen, M. E. (1994). Pharmacokinetic modeling of 2,4-dichlorophenoxyacetic acid (2,4-D) in rat and in rabbit brain following single dose administration. Toxicol. Lett., 74: 189 – 201.

Koschier, F. J. and Berndt, W. O. (1977). Evaluation of acute and short-term administration of 2,4,5-trichlorophenoxyacetate with respect to renal proximal tubular transport. *Fd Cosmet Toxicol.,* 15, 297 – 301.

Koschier, F. J., Girard, P. R., and Hong, S.K. (1978). Transport of 2,4-dichlorophenoxyacetate by rat renal cortical slices. *Toxicol. Appl. Pharmacol.,* 45, 883 – 894.

Landry, T. D., Eisenbrandt, D. L., Gushow, T. S., Phillips, J. E., and Wackerly, D. L. (1985). Triclopyr: 13-week dietary toxicity study and 4-week pharmacokinetic study in Fischer 344 rats. Toxicologist 5: 1.

Mann, W. A., Welzel, G. E., Goldstein, R. S., Sozio, R. S., Cyronak, M. J., Kao, J., and Kinter, L. B. (1991). Characterization of the renal effects and renal elimination of sulotroban in the dog. *J. Pharm. Exp. Ther.,* 259(3): 1231 – 1240.

Middendorf, P., Timchalk, C., Kropscott, B., and Rick, D. (1994). Forest worker exposure to GARLON 4 herbicide. *App. Occup. Environ. Hyg.,* 9(9): 589 – 594.

Mordenti, J. (1986). Man versus beast: pharmacokinetic scaling in mammals. *J. Pharm. Sci.,* 75(11), 1028 – 1040.

Munro, I. C., Carlo, G. L., Orr, J. C., Sund, K. G., Wilson, R. M., Kennelpohl, E., Lunch, B. S., Jablinske, M., and Lee, N. L. (1992). A comprehensive, integrated review and evaluation of the scientific evidence relating to the safety of the herbicide 2,4-D. J. Am. Coll. Toxicol., 11 (5), 559 –664.

Orberg, J. (1980). Effects of low protein consumption on the renal clearance of 2,4-dichlorophenoxyacetic acid (2,4-D) in goats. *Acta Pharmacol. et Toxicol.,* 46, 138 – 140.

Orberg, J. (1980). Observations on the 2,4-dichloropheoxyacetic acid (2,4-D) excretion in the goat. *Acta Pharmacol. et Toxicol.,* 46, 78 – 80.

Osborne, C. A., Low, D. G., and Finco, D. R. (1972). *Canine and Feline Urology,* pp. 70 – 73. Saunders, Philadelphia, PA.

Pelletier, O., Ritter, L., Caron, J. and Somers, D. (1989). Disposition of 2,4-dichlorophenoxyacetic acid salt by Fischer 344 rats dosed orally and dermally. *J. Toxicol. Environ. Health,* 28, 221 – 234.

Piper, W. N., Rose, J. Q., Leng, M. L. and Gehring, P. J. (1973). The fate of 2,4,5-trichlorophenoxyacetic acid (2,4,5-T) following oral administration to rats and dogs. *Toxicol. Appl. Pharmacol.,* 26(3), 339 – 351.

Rees, D. C. and Hattis, D. (1994). Developing quantitative strategies for animal to human extrapolation. In: *Principles and Methods of Toxicology*, 3rd Ed., (Ed. A.W. Hayes), Raven Press, N.Y., pp. 275 – 313.

Rennick, B., Hamilton, B., and Evans, R. (1961). Development of renal tubular transports of TEA and PAH in the puppy and piglet. *Am. J. Physiol.*, 201: 743 – 746.

Rowe, V.K. and Humas, T. A. (1954). Summary of toxicological information on 2,4-D and 2,4,5-T type herbicides and an evaluation of the hazards to livestock associated with their use. *Am. J. Vet. Res.*, 15, 622 – 629.

Rowland, M. and Tozer, T. N. (1996). In Clinical pharmacokinetics: concepts and applications., pp. 160 – 172. Lea & Febiger, Philadelphia, PA.

Russel, F. G. M., Wouterse, A. C., and Van Ginneken, C. A. M. (1987a). Physiologically based pharmacokinetic model for the renal clearance of phenosulfonphthalein and the interaction with probenecid and salicyluric acid in the dog. *J. Pharm. Biopharm.*, 15(4): 349 – 368.

Russel, F. G. M., Wouterse, A. C., and Van Ginneken, C. A. M. (1987b). Physiologically based pharmacokinetic model for the renal clearance of salicyluric acid and the interaction with phenolsulfonphthalein in the dog. *Drug Metab. Dispos.*, 15: 695 – 701.

Russel, F. G. M., Wouterse, A. C., and Van Ginneken, C. A. M. (1989). Physiologically based pharmacokinetic model for the renal clearance of iodopyracet and the interaction with probenecid in the dog. *Biopharm. Drug Dispos.*, 10: 137 – 152.

Sauerhoff, M. W., Braun, W. H., Blau, G. E. and Gehring, P. J. (1977). The fate of 2,4-dichlorophenoxyacetic acid (2,4-D) following oral administration to man. *Toxicology*, 8, 3 – 11.

Shuster, V. L. and Seldin, D. W. (1992). Renal clearance. In: *The Kidney: Physiology and Pathophysiology* (D.W. Seldin and G. Giebisch, Eds.), pp. 943 – 973, Raven Press, New York.

Smith, F. A., Nolan, R. J., Hermann, E. A., and Ramsey, J. C. (1980). Pharmacokinetics of 2,4-dichlorophenoxyacetic acid (2,4-D) in Fischer 344 rats. Technical Report of The Dow Chemical Company.

Timchalk, (1994). 2,4-Dichlorophenoxyacetic acid (2,4-D): pharmacokinetics in the dog. Summary methods and data, Report to Industry Task Force II on 2,4-D.

Timchalk, C. and Nolan, R. J. (1997). Pharmacokinetics of triclopyr (3,5,6-trichloro-2-pyridyloxyacetic acid) in the beagle dog and rhesus monkey: perspective on the reduced capacity of dogs to excrete this organic acid relative to rat, monkey and human. Toxicol. Appl. Pharmacol., 144, 268 – 278.

Timchalk, C., Dryzga, M. D., and Kastl, P. E. (1990). Pharmacokinetics and metabolism of triclopyr (3,5,6-trichloro-2-pyridinyloxyacetic acid) in Fischer 344 rats. Toxicology, 62: 71 – 87.

Timchalk, C., Finco, D. R. and Quast, J. F. (1997). Evaluation of renal function in rhesus monkeys and comparison to beagle dogs following oral administration of the organic acid triclopyr (3,5,6-trichloro-2-pyridinyloxyacetic acid). Fund. Appl. Toxicol., 36: 47 – 53.

Weiner, J. M. (1973). Transport of weak acids and bases. In Handbook of physiology, Section 8: renal physiology, pp. 521 – 554. American Physiology Society, Washington, DC, Williams & Wilkins Co., Baltimore, MD.

Worthing, C. R. (1987). The Pesticide Manual, 8th ed., p824. British Crop Protection Council

6 MODELING THE UPTAKE AND DISPOSITION OF HYDROPHOBIC ORGANIC CHEMICALS IN FISH USING A PHYSIOLOGICALLY BASED APPROACH

JOHN W. NICHOLS

Scientist, U.S. EPA,Research & Dev., Nat'l Health & Envirn. Effects Research Laboratory, Mid-Continent Ecology Division, Duluth, Minnesota, 55804.

Abstract: The development of physiologically based toxicokinetic (PBTK) models for hydrophobic chemicals in fish requires: 1) an understanding of chemical efflux at fish gills; 2) knowledge of the factors that limit chemical exchange between blood and tissues; and, 3) a mechanistic description of chemical uptake from the diet. Recently obtained data suggest that existing models of chemical flux at fish gills can be used to predict branchial elimination of hydrophobic compounds. Empirical relationships derived from these data are sufficient to estimate equilibrium blood:water partitioning from chemical log KOW. Empirical relationships that predict tissue:water partitioning, and by extension tissue:blood partitioning, are not as well established. Factors that limit dietary uptake of hydrophobic compounds by fish are evaluated in PBTK models for 2,3,7,8-tetrachlorodibenzo-p-dioxin (TCDD) and 2,2',5,5'-tetrachlorobiphenyl (TCB). A diffusion and/or desorption limitation appears to operate along the entire length of the fish gastrointestinal tract. This observation is consistent with earlier work which suggested that dietary assimilation efficiency declines at very high log KOW values, although more research is needed using realistic diets. The utility of this information for interpreting chemical residues in field-collected animals is discussed.

6.1 Development of PBTK Models for Fish

The use of physiologically based toxicokinetic (PBTK) models in mammalian toxicology is well established. In contrast to more conventional 'data based' models, PBTK models provide a rational basis for extrapolating among chemicals and species. Rate constants for chemical transfer among compartments are based on chemical and biological information, and the models are designed to generate predictions of the chemical time-course in specific tissues and organs. This information can then be combined with tissue effects information to provide a complete toxicological description. Mammalian PBTK modeling efforts are driven largely by the need to support human health risk assessments for chemicals, and in particular by the need to extrapolate data collected from laboratory test species to humans. In this context, there is a need to consider factors such as aging, health status,

J. Krüse, H.J.M. Verhaar, and W.K. de Raat (eds.), The Practical Applicability of Toxicokinetic Models in the Risk Assessment of Chemicals, 109-133.

and the activity of specific metabolic pathways, that could result in increased vulnerability among a subset of the human population. Idiosyncratic responses to chemicals that are of little importance from a population-based perspective attract considerable attention, prompting the need for highly detailed descriptions of chemical exposure and effect.

In contrast to human health risk assessments, ecological assessments for chemicals are typified by the need to protect a large number of potentially exposed species. Multiple exposure routes, fluctuating exposures, chemical mixtures, and complex interactions between animals and their environment complicate matters further. Because it is not possible to test all of the species and chemicals of interest, a need exists for methods to extrapolate limited testing data to a large number of untested species and chemicals, and to identify species which, for toxicokinetic or other reasons, may be particularly sensitive to important classes of environmental contaminants. The ability to incorporate species-specific information into PBTK models, and to mechanistically describe all major routes of exposure makes them well suited for this purpose also.

To date, PBTK models for fish have been developed for perhaps a dozen compounds and at least eight different species. Many of these models have been described in recent reviews (McKim and Nichols, 1994; Nichols, 1999), although new models continue to emerge. The first PBTK models for fish were adapted from rodent models and incorporated intravascular routes of exposure (Zaharko et al., 1972; Bungay et al., 1976). Later models have incorporated both the branchial (Nichols et al., 1990) and dermal (Nichols et al., 1996) routes of exposure. PBTK models for fish have been used to describe the uptake and disposition of waterborne chemicals of low to intermediate hydrophobicity ($1.5 < \log KOW < 4.5$), and to extrapolate this data among species (McKim and Nichols, 1994). Presently, it is possible to predict the kinetics of moderately hydrophobic compounds from knowledge of cardiovascular and respiratory function, and empirical relationships between chemical partitioning and log KOW, provided that they do not undergo substantial metabolic biotransformation. Additional efforts have been made to incorporate metabolism into PBTK models for fish and to relate dosimetry information to toxic effects in specific tissues (Law et al., 1991; Abbas and Hayton, 1997).

As chemical hydrophobicity increases, the importance of dietary uptake relative to uptake directly from water also tends to increase. The point at which dietary uptake begins to predominate undoubtedly varies with a number of factors; however, it is generally accepted that the diet is the principal route of exposure for chemicals with log KOW values greater than about 5 (Bruggeman et al., 1984). Hydrophobic organic compounds continue to attract attention because of their toxicity, persistence and tendency to accumulate in aquatic biota.

The purpose of this presentation is to describe recent efforts to develop PBTK models for the uptake and disposition of hydrophobic organic chemicals in fish. Emphasis is placed on understanding chemical elimination at fish gills, factors that limit chemical exchange between blood and tissues, and the development of a mechanistic dietary uptake description. Specific points are Illustrated by describing PBTK models for 2,3,7,8-tetachlorodibenzo-p-dioxin (TCDD) and 2,2',5,5'-tetrachlorobiphenyl (TCB). Potential uses for these models and the information that derives from them are also discussed.

6.2 Branchial Efflux of Organic Chemicals

For many high log KOW compounds, the gills probably represent a route of chemical elimination. This is because the processes that accompany digestion of a meal, including a reduction in volume and uptake of dietary lipid, increase the inward gradient for chemical diffusion in the gastrointestinal (GI) tract (Connolly and Pederson, 1988; Gobas et al., 1988, 1993, 1999). A potential result of this enhanced uptake is that chemical concentrations in fish may be greater than those of their prey (corrected for differences in lipid content) and higher than those expected from equilibrium partitioning between the fish and surrounding water. Under these circumstances, branchial efflux tends to restore an equilibrium distribution of chemical, and the rate of efflux, relative to that of dietary uptake, can impact the extent to which chemicals will ultimately accumulate.

6.2.1 Erickson-McKim Gill Models

Erickson and McKim (1990 a,b) developed a pair of mechanistic models to describe the branchial uptake of waterborne organic chemicals by fish. In the first model (Erickson and McKim, 1990a) uptake was limited only by the capacity of water to deliver chemical to the gills and the capacity of blood to remove chemical from the gills. Measured and predicted uptake rates, as a function of chemical log KOW, are plotted in Figure 1. The second model was expanded to include the possibility of kinetic limitations due to diffusion and chemical binding to dissolved organic material (DOC, termed 'high molecular weight organic matter' by Erickson and McKim, 1990b). The extent of DOC binding was estimated as a function of chemical log KOW using the relationship given by McCarthy and Jimenez (1985). Importantly, McCarthy and Jimenez (1985) reported that the dissociation kinetics of DOC-bound chemical were slow relative to the residence time of water at fish gills. In the

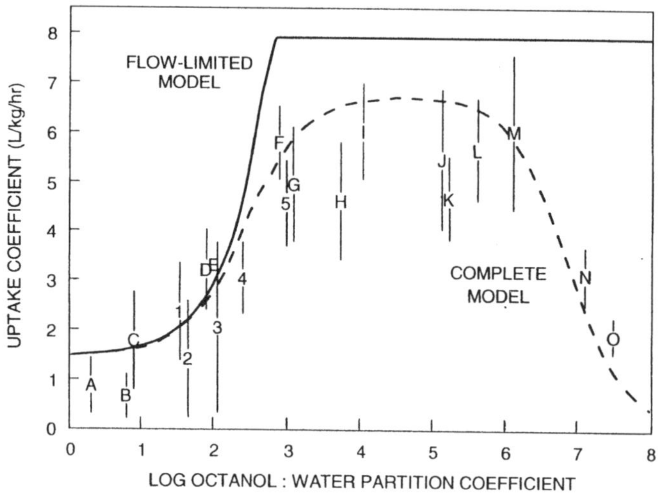

Figure 1. Observed and predicted relationship of gill uptake rate to octanol:water partitioning. Data from sublethal exposures are denoted by A - ethyl formate; B - ethyl acetate; C - 1-butanol; D - nitrobenzene; E - p-cresol; F - chlorobenzene; G - 2,4-dichlorophenol; H - 2,4,5-trichlorophenol; I - 1-decanol; J - 1-dodecanol; K - pentachlorophenol; L - hexachlorobenzene; M - 2,2',5,5'-tetrachlorobiphenyl; N - fenvalerate; and O - mirex. Lethal exposures are denoted by 1 - benzaldehyde; 2 - 2,4-dinitrophenol; 3 - MS-222; 4 - malathion; 5 - 1-octanol. The solid shows the prediction of a flow-limited gill model. The dashed line shows the prediction of a gill model with diffusion limitations and strong binding to DOC (adapted from Erickson and McKim, 1990b).

expanded gill model, Erickson and McKim (1990b) assumed that only chemicals dissolved in water were available to diffuse across branchial cell membranes. Additional calculations suggested that diffusional resistances would lower the rate of uptake by about 15% from the maximum defined by water flow. The complete model predicted an observed decline in branchial uptake of chemicals with KOW values greater than 6 (Figure 1). This decline in uptake is important because it contributes to the shift from branchial uptake to dietary uptake for such compounds.

6.2.2 Empirical Relationship Between Log PBW and Log KOW

The expanded Erickson-McKim (1990b) model makes two additional assumptions with respect to branchial flux that could impact it's utility for high log KOWcompounds: 1) branchial flux proceeds to equilibrium between dissolved chemical concentrations in the exchanging blood and water flows; and, 2) the kinetics of chemical dissociation from binding elements in blood, in contrast to DOC binding, are relatively fast so that the ratio of bound to free chemical is approximately at equilibrium at all points within the blood. With these assumptions, the gradient for chemical diffusion can be expressed as:

$$C_{INSPIRED\ WATER} - C_{AFFERENT\ BLOOD}\ P_{BW} \qquad (1)$$

where the chemical concentrations in blood and water refer to dissolved chemical, and PBW is the equilibrium blood:water partition coefficient.

Other parameters in the model contribute to determining the rate of branchial flux. Unlike PBW, however, these parameters (e.g., cardiac output, effective respiratory volume, surface area for diffusion) vary little if at all with chemical log KOW.

Using an in vitro headspace technique and blood from rainbow trout, Hoffman et al. (1992) estimated PBW values for several chemicals with log KOW values up to about 4.5. Similar observations were then made using blood from several other fish species (Bertelsen et al., 1998). For any given species, a plot of log PBW vs. log KOW gives a linear relationship (Figure 2a). Using these empirical relationships as inputs to the gill model it has been possible to predict the observed branchial flux of compounds exhibiting low to moderate hydrophobicity (Nichols et al., 1991). Until recently, however, there has been some question whether branchial efflux of high log KOWcompounds could be predicted using the simplifying assumptions of the gill model and linear extrapolations of these partitioning relationships.

Data collected by Fitzsimmons et al. (2001) now permit a direct assessment of branchial efflux for high log KOW compounds. In these studies, rainbow trout were dosed with a series PCBs with log KOW values ranging from 5.8 to 8.2. The trout were placed in respirometer-metabolism chambers and a large volume expired water was passed through a column filled with Ambersorb® resin. The resin was then extracted and the PCBs were quantitated by GC/MS. Chemical concentrations in expired water were found to be in the nanomolar concentration range. Measured values in blood and water were sufficient, however, to calculate apparent PBW values. In effect, the Erickson-McKim model was used to calculate PBW values that would have been required to explain observed rates of elimination, adopting all model assumptions. These values were then compared to the empirical relationship established previously for rainbow trout using in vitro partitioning data (Bertelsen et al., 1998). The data collected by Fitzsimmon et al. (2001) yielded a linear relationship between log PBW and log KOW (Figure 2a) with slope and intercept terms statistically indistinguishable from those calculated for lower log KOW compounds. Combining all data, a linear relationship was obtained that can be used to predict partitioning for compounds with log KOWvalues ranging from 1.5 to greater than 8 (Figure 2b).

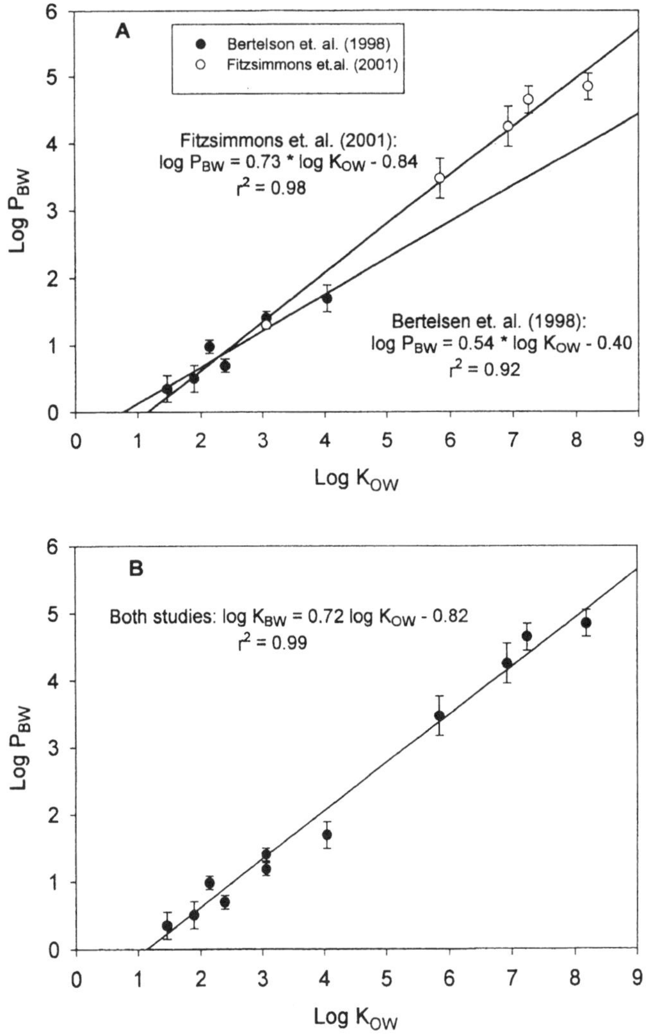

Figure 2. Empirical relationship between blood:water and octanol:water partitioning. A. Linear regressions of log PBW vs. log KOW were derived using in vitro partitioning data reported by Bertelsen et al. (1998) for rainbow trout and apparent PBWvalues provided by Fitzsimmons et al. (2001). B. Linear regression using data from all studies with trout (adapted from Fitzsimmons et al., 2001).

6.3 Chemical Distribution between Blood and Tissues

6.3.1 Equilibrium Tissue:Blood Partitioning.

In the 1980s, rapid progress in the development and use of mammalian PBTK models was facilitated by the development of in vitro methods to estimate tissue:blood partition coefficients for volatile compounds (Gargas et al., 1989). These techniques were subsequently used to estimate tissue:blood partitioning for volatile compounds in fish (Hoffman et al., 1992). Historically, PBTK models for non-volatile compounds have depended on the existence of steady-state exposure data from which to estimate partitioning relationships. Although several partitioning systems have been developed for use with non-volatile compounds (Jepson et al., 1994; Murphy et al., 1995; Abbas and Hayton, 1997), the number of non-volatiles for which in vitro partitioning estimates have been obtained remains relatively small.

In recent years, several research groups have published tissue composition- based and/or empirical methods to estimate tissue:blood partitioning values. The composition-based approach is founded on the premise that tissue:blood partitioning can be estimated from the relative content of materials (e.g., neutral lipid, phospholipids, protein and water) in tissue and blood that contribute to this partitioning. Chemical distribution to lipid and water is generally assumed to follow directly from octanol:water partioning (or partitioning in some other comparable system), while chemical affinity for other tissue constituents is expressed as a fraction of that attributed to lipid (Poulin and Krishan, 1995, 1996).

Alternatively, if sufficient data exist it is possible to use an empirical approach that does not depend on assumed relationships between octanol:water partitioning and partitioning to tissue constituents (DeJongh et al., 1997; Bertelsen et al., 1998). Using data from several fish species, Bertelsen et al., (1998) regressed tissue:water partitioning values against chemical log KOW and tissue lipid content to derive a series of tissue-specific empirical relationships. Chemical log KOW was shown to be a good predictor of tissue:water partitioning in all tissues, and a generalized equation was provided relating tissue:water partitioning to log Kow and tissue lipid content (Figure 3). An evaluation of fitted slope and intercept terms for individual tissues suggested, however, that partitioning to non-lipid material contributes substantially to chemical affinity in lean tissues. More importantly, fitted slope terms differed among tissues (including blood). This result suggests that tissue:blood partitioning, estimated from the ratio of tissue:water and blood:water values, will vary systematically with chemical log KOW.

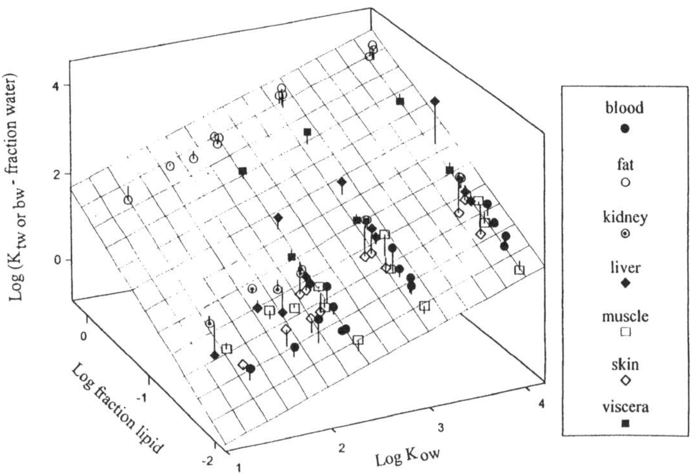

Figure 3. Partition coefficient response surface predicted from chemical log KOW and log total lipid content. Individual points are the residuals of predicted values for the combined model using log KOW and log total lipid content as descriptors of partitioning, after correcting for water content (from Bertelsen et al., 1998).

The need for empirical and semi-empirical partitioning models depends on the desired accuracy of PBTK model predictions. Lipid content is the major determinant of tissue partitioning for hydrophobic compounds, and the ratio of total lipid in a tissue to that in blood is often sufficient to estimate the steady-state tissue:blood chemical concentration ratio within a factor of 2 to 3 (Nichols et al., 1998). For many applications, this level of accuracy is sufficient. In other cases, specific binding has a large impact on the disposition of hydrophobic compounds and their metabolic products (Bergman et al., 1982; Poland et al., 1989; Bergman et al., 1994). It may be possible to develop structure-activity relationships (SARs) for different types of binding that could be incorporated into predictive partitioning models. Partitioning information for a large number of compounds would be required, however, to evaluate and refine these approaches.

6.3.2 Flow vs. Diffusion Limitations

The development of a PBTK model requires that assumptions be made about factors that limit chemical flux between blood and tissues. The simplest formulation assumes that chemical flux proceeds to equilibrium during the time available for chemical exchange. Under these circumstances blood flow rate to the tissue controls the rate of chemical accumulation, and the chemical concentration in blood exiting the tissue is a simple function of that in the tissue and a tissue:blood partition coefficient. Remarkably, this simplifying assumption has been shown to adequately predict the observed kinetics of a large number of compounds in both fish and mammals.

The present focus on hydrophobic compounds requires, however, that consideration be given to possible diffusion limitations on chemical flux. Mammalian PBTK models for PCBs, TCDD and other high molecular weight halogenated compounds often incorporate diffusion limitations in one or more tissues to account for observed rates of chemical accumulation (Andersen et al., 1993; Kedderis et al., 1993). Mass-balance equations are written for both the blood and extravascular tissue spaces and permeability coefficients are used to relate chemical flux to the magnitude of the concentration gradient. These coefficients have been interpreted as the product of a true diffusion coefficient and the effective surface area for exchange; however, efforts to independently estimate these two parameters are rare. Blood perfusion rates to tissues are generally lower in fish than in mammals, but the impact of this difference is difficult to predict. Although lower blood flow rates may increase the residence time of blood in tissue, this increase may be accompanied by lower capillary densities, increasing the diffusion distance.

6.4 PBTK Models for Fish

In this section PBTK models for TCDD and TCB are described as a means of illustrating points made previously. Both models incorporate mathematical descriptions of chemical uptake from the diet. In the TCDD model, a relatively simple gut description is used to evaluate competing assumptions about factors that limit dietary uptake. The purpose of the TCB model was to develop a detailed description of dietary uptake and to relate observed kinetics to aspects of fish gastrointestinal physiology.

6.5 TCDD Model

A PBTK model was developed to describe the accumulation of TCDD in chronic dietary exposures with brook trout (Nichols et al., 1998). Special emphasis was placed on describing the maternal transfer of TCDD to developing ovaries, as toxic effects on fish are thought to be exerted during early development. The exposure itself was described by Tietge et al. (1998) and toxic effects on fry derived from TCDD-dosed adults were described by Johnson et al. (1998). Briefly, the study consisted of a 28-d loading phase, a 77-d maintenance phase, and a 77-d spawning/depuration phase. The exposure was carried out by spiking [3H] - TCDD into a prepared diet. Average TCDD concentrations in the loading diet ranged from 733 to 10,555 pg/g.

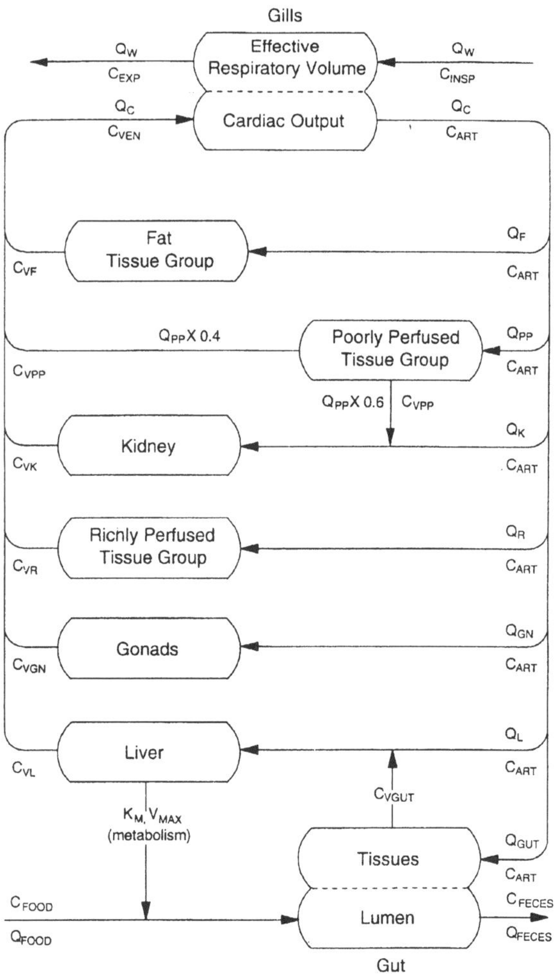

Figure 4. Schematic representation of a physiologically based toxicokinetic model for dietary uptake of 2,3,7,8-tetrachlorodibenzo-p-dioxin by brook trout (adapted from Nichols et al., 1998). QW - effective respiratory volume; QC - cardiac output; CINSP - chemical concentration in inspired water; CEXP - chemical concentration in expired water; CART - chemical concentration in arterial blood; QF, QPP, QK, QR, QGN, QL, QGUT - blood flow to the fat, poorly perfused, kidney, richly perfused, gonad, liver and gut compartments; CVF, CVPP, CVK, CVR, CVGN, CVL, CVGUT - chemical concentrations in blood exiting the fat, poorly perfused, kidney, richly perfused, gonad, liver and gut compartments; CVEN - chemical concentration in mixed venous blood; CFOOD - chemical concentration in food; QFOOD - feeding rate expressed as a bulk flow rate; CFECES - chemical concentration in feces; QFECES - fecal production rate; VMAX, KM - metabolic rate and capacity parameters.

Dose levels were then reduced by a factor of about 7 to 8 in an effort to achieve constant whole- body concentrations during the maintenance phase. This experimental design provided an opportunity to examine TCDD kinetics during a period of rapid accumulation, followed by a near steady-state condition and, finally, depuration.

The TCDD model is shown in Figure 4. Many of the physiological and anatomical inputs were obtained from studies of brook trout. Others, including blood flow rates to tissues, were set equal to those of rainbow trout. Tissue:blood partitioning was determined from concentration ratios in tissues when fish were at or near steady- state. Blood:water partitioning was estimated by extrapolation of the relationship given by Bertelsen et al. (1998).

Two different sub-models were developed to describe TCDD uptake from the diet The first, termed a 'fecal partitioning' sub-model, was based upon the assumption that a chemical equilibrium is established between feces (CFEC) and blood exiting the intestinal tract (CVGT):

$$C_{FEC} = C_{VGT}\ P_{FEC:B} \qquad (2)$$

where PFEC:B is the feces:blood equilibrium chemical partition coefficient. This approach is similar to that used by Barber et al. (1991) in a model for lake trout, the principal difference being that equilibrium is established with venous blood exiting the gut and not with the whole fish. From mass-balance considerations it follows that:

$$Q_{FOOD}\ C_{FOOD} - Q_{FEC}\ C_{FEC} = Q_{GT}\ C_{VGT} - Q_{GT}\ C_{ART} \qquad (3)$$

where QFOOD is the feeding rate, QFEC equals the fecal egestion rate, QGT is the blood flow rate to the intestines, CFOOD equals the TCDD concentration in the diet, and CART is the chemical concentration in arterial blood. Substituting Eq. 2 into Eq. 3 and solving for CVGT yields:

$$C_{VGT} = (Q_{GT}\ C_{ART} + Q_{FOOD}\ C_{FOOD})/(Q_{GT} + Q_{FEC}\ P_{FEC:B}) \qquad (4)$$

A second dietary uptake description was developed from the assumption that kinetic limitations prevent a chemical equilibrium between blood and feces. It was assumed that this limitation exhibits first-order kinetics with respect to the chemical concentration in feces. The 'diffusion-limited' sub-model includes mass-balance differential equations for both the contents of the intestinal tract and the tissues. For the feces:

$$dA_{FEC}/dt = Q_{FOOD}\ C_{FOOD} - Q_{FEC}\ C_{FEC} - K_{GT}\ (C_{FEC} - C_{GT}\ P_{FEC:GT}) \qquad (5)$$

where AFEC is the amount of TCDD in feces, KGT is a first order rate constant, CGT is the chemical concentration in gut tissues, and PFEC:GT is the feces:gut tissue equilibrium chemical partition coefficient. For the tissues of the intestinal tract:

$$dA_{GT}/dt = Q_{GT}(C_{ART} - C_{VGT}) + K_{GT}(C_{FEC} - C_{GT}\,P_{FEC:GT}) \tag{6}$$

The chemical concentration in venous blood draining the gut is then determined from that of the gut tissues using a gut tissue:blood partition coefficient:

$$dA_{GT}/dt = Q_{GT}(C_{ART} - C_{VGT}) + K_{GT}(C_{FEC} - C_{GT}\,P_{FEC:GT}) \tag{7}$$

In this description, chemical flux across the GI tract is diffusion-limited when KGT < QGT. Model parameterization and the procedure for estimating KGT were given by Nichols et al. (1998).

Attempts to simulate TCDD accumulation using the fecal partitioning assumption resulted in overestimation of observed chemical assimilation from the diet (net assimilation, determined from chemical residues in fish) and elimination rates faster than those observed during the depuration phase of the study (Figure 5).

Good agreement of model predictions with measured whole-body residues and dietary assimilation estimates was obtained by using the diffusion-limited gut description and fitting the value of KGT. The value of KGT that gave the best correspondence between measured and predicted residues was about 5% of QGT.

TCDD residues in all tissues except fat were adequately simulated by assuming that chemical distribution to tissues was blood flow-limited. Model predictions of chemical accumulation in fat were improved by imposing a diffusion limitation on chemical flux. The best fit to the data was obtained by limiting the uptake rate to about 25% of that calculated using a flow-limited description. Figure 6 shows model simulations and observed TCDD residues in selected tissues. Despite rapid tissue growth and changes in chemical affinity, an equilibrium between the ovaries and blood was attained early in the loading phase of the study. This observation is important because it suggests that chemical concentrations in whole fish would suffice to estimate TCDD concentrations in eggs, provided that partitioning relationships were known. Interestingly, spawning resulted in a modest increase in whole-body TCDD concentration. In this respect, brook trout resemble lake trout, another member of the charr family. Miller (1993) found that lake trout invest a relatively small proportion of their somatic lipid stores in each spawn and as a result eliminate a small percentage of their whole-body chemical burden by this route.

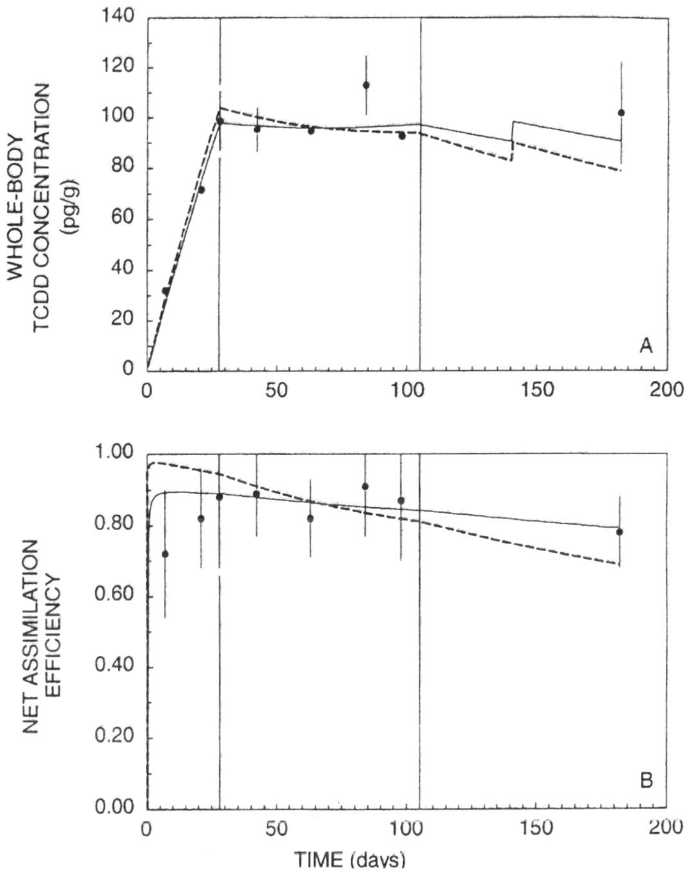

Figure 5. Accumulation of 2,3,7,8-tetrachlorodibenzo-p-dioxin (TCDD) in brook trout. Measured whole-body concentrations (mean and calculated assimilation efficiencies are shown as individual points. Simulations were obtained using a physiologically based toxicokinetic model for brook trout (Nichols et al., 1998). Dashed lines were generated using a 'fecal partitioning' gut sub-model. Solid lines were obtained by imposing a 'diffusion limitation' on dietary uptake (redrawn from Nichols et al., 1998).

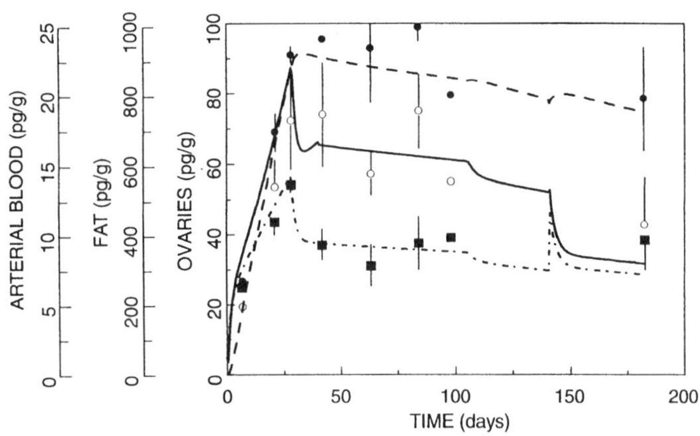

Figure 6. Time-course of 2,3,7,8-tetrachlorodibenzo-p-dioxin (TCDD) in fat, ovaries and blood of brook trout during a chronic feeding study. Data are from fish exposed to 733 pg/g in the loading dose. Simulated chemical residues are shown as dotted (blood), dashed (ovaries), and solid (fat) lines. Measure residues (mean ± SD) are shown as dots (fat), open circles (ovaries), and solid squares (blood)(redrawn from Nichols et al., 1998).

6.6 TCB Model

Subsequent to the TCDD study we developed a PBTK model for dietary uptake of TCB. The goal of this effort was to develop a detailed description of the gut, and in particular to examine factors that control the rate and extent of dietary uptake. The model was developed and evaluated using data from feeding studies with TCB (Nichols et al., 2001). Subadult (75 - 125 g) rainbow trout were fed 60 d-old fathead minnows which had been exposed previously to [14C] - TCB in water. Feeding rates and TCB concentrations in minnows were designed to simulate an "environmentally relevant" dietary exposure. Trout were killed 6, 12, 24, 48, or 96 h after consuming a meal of contaminated minnows. Those killed at 96 hr were fed a meal of uncontaminated minnows at 48 h. The GI tract of each fish was partitioned into the stomach, upper intestine (excluding pyloric ceca) and lower intestine, and TCB concentrations were measured in gut contents and tissues, as well as in other selected tissues. In supporting studies, we also examined the pattern of gastric evacuation and changes in the wet weight, dry weight, and lipid content of digesta as it moved down the GI tract.

A schematic of the dietary uptake sub-model for TCB is given in Figure 7. Symbols and subscripts are defined in Table 1. The structure of this model is based on the anatomy and physiology of the fish GI tract, and parameter values that pertain to the flow and processing of the meal were

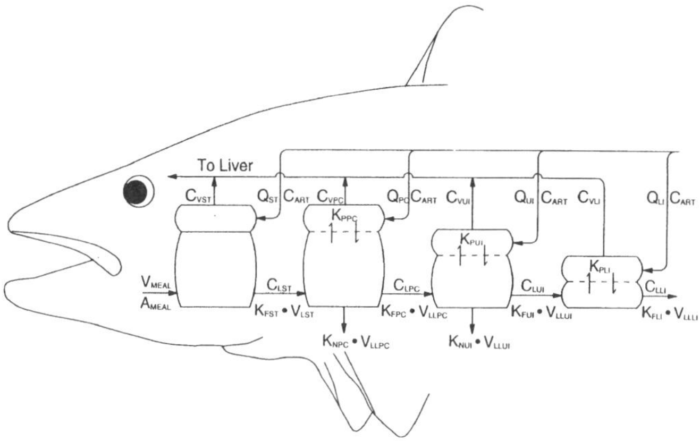

Figure 7. Physiologically based sub-model used to describe dietary uptake of 2,2',5,5'- tetrachlorobiphenyl (TCB) by rainbow trout. Symbols and subscripts are defined in Table 1.

determined by modeling to observed changes in the wet weight and lipid content of digesta. Gastric emptying was described using an exponential function. Lumenal volumes of the pyloric ceca, upper intestine and lower intestine were simulated using first-order relationships to describe nutrient absorption (pyloric ceca and upper intestine only) and the bulk flow of digesta from one compartment to the next.

From mass-balance considerations, the rate of change of the amount of chemical within tissues of the pyloric ceca, upper intestine and lower intestine was set equal the blood flow rate to the tissue times the arterial-to-venous difference in chemical concentration, plus the diffusive exchange with the corresponding lumenal sub-compartment:

$$dA_{TI}/dt = Q_I (C_A - C_{VI}) + K_{PI}\, SA_I (C_{LI} - C_{TI}\, P_{LI:TI}) \qquad (8)$$

where the chemical concentration in the tissue is calculated as,

$$C_{TI} = A_{TI}/V_{TI} \qquad (9)$$

the concentration in venous blood exiting the tissue is given as,

$$C_{VI} = C_{TI}/P_{TI:B} \qquad (10)$$

and the subscript (I) refers to the gut segment of interest.

The direction and magnitude of the diffusion gradient is determined by the difference in chemical activity between the lumenal contents and the corresponding gut tissues, referenced to each tissue using a lumen:tissue parti-

Table 1. Definitions of Terms Used in a Dietary Uptake Model for TCB.

V_{TI}	Volume of the tissue
V_{LI}	Volume of the lumenal contents
V_{LLI}	Volume of the lumenal contents exceeding a predetermined "baseline" value
A_{TI}	Amount of chemical in the tissue
A_{LI}	Amount of chemical in the lumenal contents
C_{TI}	Concentration of chemical in the tissue
C_{LI}	Concentration of chemical in the lumenal contents
C_{VI}	Concentration of chemical in venous blood from the tissue
S_{AI}	Surface area for chemical diffusion
K_{PI}	Fitted first-order permeability coefficient for gut tissue gut lumen chemical diffusion
	KNI Fitted first-order constant for reduction in lumenal volume due to nutrient uptake
	KFI Fitted first-order constant for reduction in lumenal volume due bulk flow of digesta out of the (I) lumenal compartment
Q_I	ARTERIAL BLOOD FLOW TO THE TISSUE
$P_{L:I}$	Lumen:tissue equilibrium partition coefficient
$P_{I:B}$	Tissue:blood equilibrium partition coefficient

Where the subscript I denotes:

ST = stomach
PC = pyloric ceca
UI = upper intestine
LI = lower intestine

A_{DOSE}	Amount of chemical in the meal
V_{DOSE}	Volume of the meal
C_A	Chemical concentration in arterial blood
K_{STA}	Fitted first-order constant for reduction in chemical mass in the stomach lumen

tion coefficient (PLI:TI). Diffusion rate constants for each gut segment were calculated as the product of the surface area for diffusion (SAI) and a permeability constant (KPI), that represents the combined resistance of the intervening diffusion barriers.

Following Bungay et al. (1981), mass-balance equations for lumenal contents of the pyloric ceca, upper intestine and lower intestine include terms for input from the upstream compartment (LI -1), egestion to the downstream compartment or to the environment, and diffusive flux into or out of the corresponding tissue sub-compartment:

$$dA_{LI}/dt = Q_{LI-1}\,C_{LI-1} - Q_{LI}\,C_{LI} + K_{PI}\,SA_I\,(C_{LI} - C_{TI}\,P_{LI:TI}) \qquad (11)$$

where,

$$C_{LI} = A_{LI} / V_{LI} \tag{12}$$

Once formulated, the gut description was imbedded within an established model for inhalation exposure (Nichols et al., 1990). In feeding studies with TCB the gills served as a route of chemical elimination. Branchial efflux was described using the Erickson-McKim (1990b) gill model, and the blood:water partition coefficient was taken from the relationship given by Fitzsimmons et al. (2001). Preliminary studies suggested that there was a modest diffusion limitation on chemical accumulation by the poorly perfused compartment (primarily white muscle) equivalent to a two-thirds reduction in tissue blood flow rate. Uptake by all other tissues was assumed to be blood flow- limited. Tissue:blood partition coefficients were determined from chemical concentration ratios in fish that were close to steady-state.

The performance of this model is shown in Figures 8 - 11. It will be noted in Figures 8 - 10 that there are no data for the pyloric ceca. The pyloric ceca are blind diverticula that branch off from the upper intestine just below the stomach. The model simulates chemical concentrations in the pyloric ceca; indeed, chemical uptake from this segment has a large impact on chemical kinetics in downstream compartments. Unfortunately, the fine diameter of the pyloric ceca makes them very difficult to sample. The kinetic behavior of this compartment must be inferred, therefore, from differences in volume,

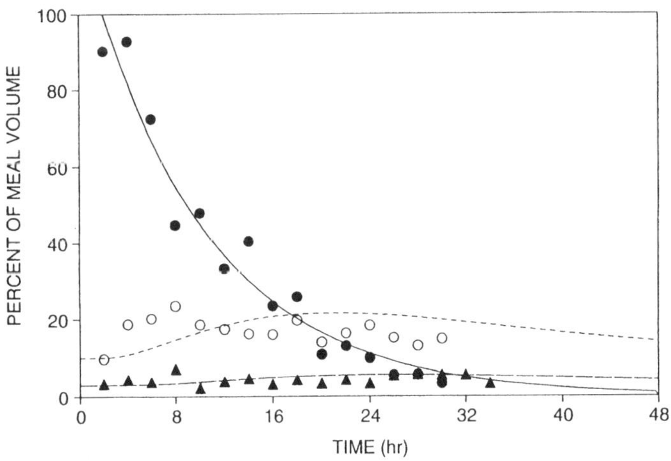

Figure 8. Changes in the wet weight of digesta in the stomach (dots), upper intestine (open circles) and lower intestine (triangles) of rainbow trout fed a single meal of fathead minnows. Measured values are given as individual points (mean ± SE). Optimized model simulations are shown as solid (stomach), small dashed (upper intestine), and large dashed (lower intestine) lines.

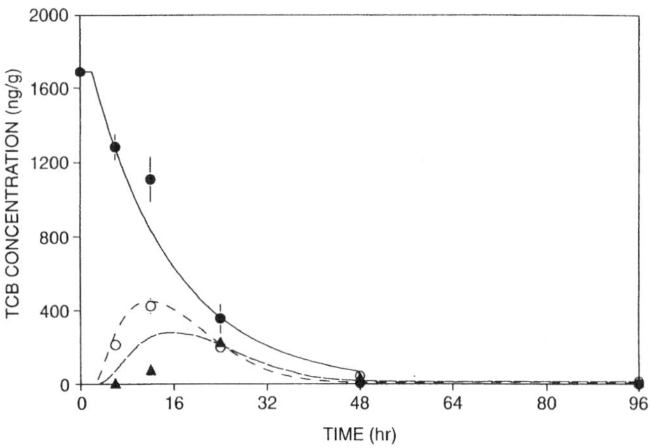

Figure 9. Time-course of 2,2',5,5'-tetrachlorobiphenyl (TCB) in contents of the stomach (dots), upper intestine (open circles) and lower intestine (triangles) of rainbow trout fed a single meal of TCB-contaminated fathead minnows. Measured values are given as individual points (mean ± SE). Optimized model simulations are shown as solid (stomach), small dashed (upper intestine), and large dashed (lower intestine) lines.

lipid content and chemical concentration in the stomach and in the upper intestine distal to the pyloric ceca (here termed "upper intestine"). Figure 8 shows the pattern of gastric evacuation and changes in the volume of digesta in both the upper and lower intestine. A notable feature of these data is the dampening of volume changes in both the upper and lower intestine. Fitted rate constants for nutrient uptake and bulk flow down the GI tract yield the model simulations shown in Figure 8 and result in an egested fecal volume equal to about 20% of the meal volume.

Figure 9 shows the simulated and observed TCB concentrations in contents of the three sampled gut segments. Importantly, the fitted rate constants that provided the best simulations of the data were essentially the same for all absorbing segments (Table 2). Chemical kinetics in the lower intestine

Table 2. Fitted first-order rate constants for evacuation of TCB from the stomach, bulk flow of digesta, and changes in lumenal volume due to nutrient uptake (hr^{-1}).

Gastric evacuation of TCB		K_{STA}	0.17
Bulk flow	Stomach ↔ pyloric ceca	K_{FST}	0.10
	Pyloric ceca ↔ upper intestine	K_{FPC}	0.05
	Upper intestine ↔ lower intestine	K_{FUI}	0.05
	Lower intestine ↔ environment	KFLI	0.25
Nutrient uptake	Pyloric ceca ↔ fish	K_{NPC}	0.15
	Upper intestine ↔ fish	K_{NUI}	0.02

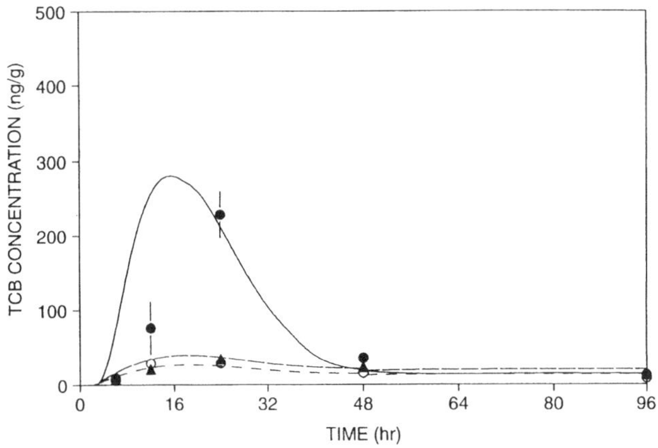

Figure 10. Time-course of 2,2',5,5'-tetrachlorobiphenyl (TCB) in arterial blood (open circles), and in the tissues (triangles) and contents (dots) of the lower intestine. Measured values are given as individual points (mean ± SE). Optimized model simulations are shown as solid (lower intestinal contents), small dashed (blood), and large dashed (lower intestinal tissues) lines.

are shown in Figure 10. The conclusion that can be drawn from these data is that the contents of the lower intestine are not in chemical equilibrium with the tissues. The tissues, on the other hand, appear to be in equilibrium

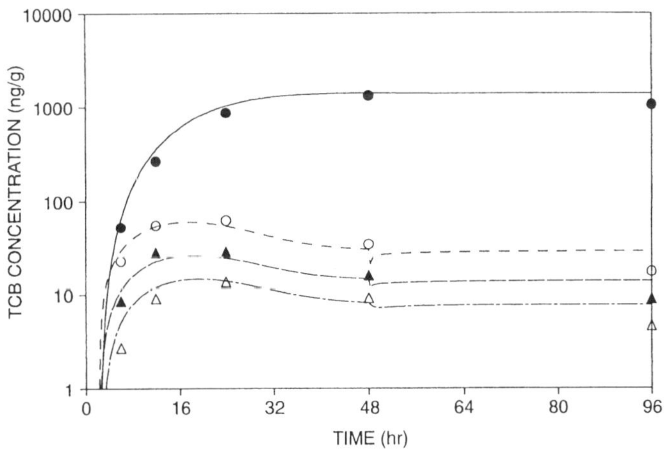

Figure 11. Time-course of 2,2',5,5'-tetrachlorobiphenyl (TCB) in the fat (dots), blood (solid triangles), liver (open circles) and muscle (open triangles) of trout fed a single meal of TCB-contaminated fathead minnows. Measured values are given as individual points (mean ± SE). optimized model simulations are shown as solid (fat), small dashed (liver), large dashed (blood), and dot-dashed (muscle) lines.

with blood. These data do not support the fecal partitioning assumption proposed earlier to describe chemical uptake from the gut.

Finally, after fitting uptake rate constants for TCB, the model was used to simulate chemical kinetics in various tissues. Figure 11 shows simulated and measured values in fat, blood, liver and muscle. The model accurately simulated the chemical time-course in all tissues, including the observed redistribution of TCB from lean tissues to fat.

6.7 Discussion

The purpose of this paper was to review recent progress on the development of PBTK models for hydrophobic organic chemicals in fish. Special attention was given to chemical elimination across fish gills, factors that limit exchange between blood and tissues, and improvements in our understanding of chemical uptake from the diet. Data collected in branchial efflux studies with high log KOW compounds provide support for the mechanistic gill model developed by Erickson and McKim (1990b). These data also yield an improved empirical relationship between log PBW and chemical log KOW that can be used to estimate PBW values across a wide range of log KOW values. Tissue and blood lipid content can be used to estimate steady-state tissue:blood partitioning of high log KOW compounds within a factor of 2 to 3 of observed values, provided that they do not exhibit specific binding. Modest improvements on lipid-based partitioning estimates can be achieved using empirical and semi-empirical partitioning models, particularly for lean tissues.

In modeling studies with fish, diffusion limitations have been indicated for chemical accumulation in fat (TCDD) and muscle (TCB). These diffusion limitations were only discernable, however, within hours of starting an exposure or during periods of rapid chemical accumulation. For exposures lasting weeks or months they are unlikely to be important. A kinetic limitation on chemical uptake appears to operate along the entire length of the fish gastrointestinal tract, the identity of which is unknown. Factors that could limit chemical flux in the GI tract include diffusion across aqueous barriers within the intestinal lumen and desorption of chemical bound to chyme and feces.

The importance of these findings is related to two, overlapping questions: 1) what determines the amount of chemical consumed by a fish that will remain associated with the animal; and 2) what determines the extent to which fish will accumulate hydrophobic compounds in an environmental setting. Previously, Gobas et al. (1988) summarized dietary assimilation data from a number of studies. Shown in Figure 12, these data suggested that dietary assimilation efficiency declines with chemical hydrophobicity at log KOW

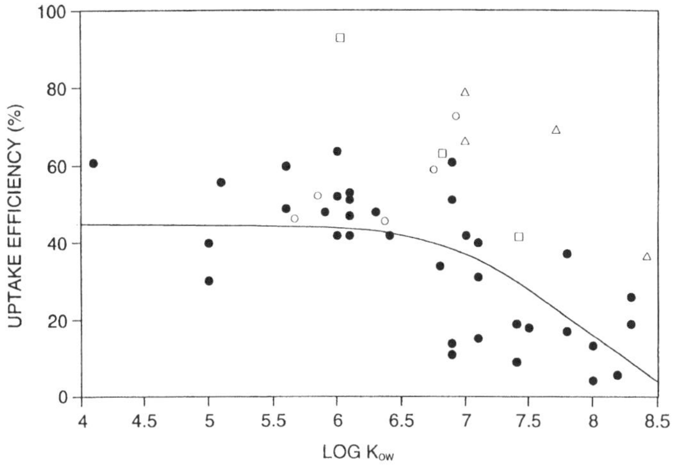

Figure 12. Observed and predicted relationship between chemical log KOW and dietary assimilation efficiency in fish. Values summarized by Gobas et al. (1988) are shown as dots. Estimates obtained by Burreau et al. (1997) are given as open circles (polychlorinated biphenyls), squares (polybrominated diphenyl ethers) and triangles (polychlorinated naphthalenes). The solid line was calculated using the fugacity model presented by Gobas et al. (1988).

values greater than about 6. Based on this observation, Gobas et al. (1988) concluded that dietary uptake is controlled by a diffusion resistance and that the magnitude of this resistence increases at high log KOWvalues. Assimilation efficiencies measured by Burreau et al., (1997) are also shown in Figure 12. In this study, northern pike were fed rainbow trout which had previously been injected with the test chemicals. Assimilation efficiencies measured by Burreau et al. (1997) are generally higher than those reported by Gobas et al. (1988) and do not exhibit a declining trend with chemical hydrophobicity. It should be noted, however, that the compounds tested by Burreau et al. (1997) represent three different chemical classes. Examined independently, data from two of the three chemical classes exhibit a decline in assimilation efficiency with chemical log KOW. The results of our work with TCB and TCDD support the conclusion that chemical assimilation from a natural diet is more efficient than previously appreciated. Nevertheless, a diffusion and/or desorption limitation appears to control absorption of these compounds in the GI tract. Additional work is required to fully understand the underlying basis, extent and log KOWdependence of this kinetic limitation.

Finally, it is important to consider dietary uptake in the context of a general need to understand the accumulation of hydrophobic organic chemicals by fish. Figure 13 shows the linear relationship between chemical accumulation and log KOW published by Mackay (1982) using data from water-only exposures. Our present understanding of chemical flux at fish gills suggests that this relationship will approximate chemical accumulation by fish at log KOW values up to about 5. Branchial flux across this range of log KOW values dominates total uptake during the initial period of accumulation and, at steady-state, the enhanced uptake that could occur from dietary sources is more than offset by chemical elimination at the gills. The factors that control accumulation of high log KOW compounds are less well known. In Figure 13 a dotted line shows the possible effect of growth dilution on whole-fish residues. A dashed line shows the potential impact of biomagnification due

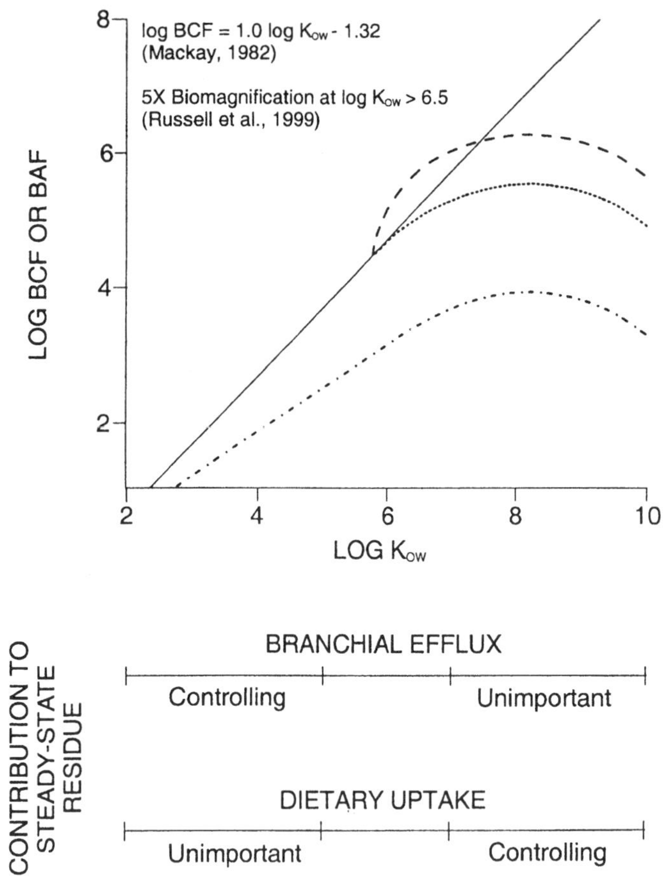

Figure 13. Hypothetical relationships between chemical accumulation in fish and log KOW. The solid line denotes the linear relationship between log BCF and log KOW given by Mackay (1982). Additional lines illustrate potential effects of growth dilution (dotted), residue biomagnification (dashed) and metabolic biotransformation (dot-dash). The maximum extent of biomagnification is similar to that observed by Russell et al. (1999). Assuming an absence of metabolism, the contributions of branchial efflux and dietary uptake to steady-state residues in fish are shown at the bottom of the figure as rough functions of chemical log KOW.

Table 3. Fitted permeability coefficients for TCB uptake (cm hr^{-1}).

Pyloric ceca lumen ↔ tissue	K_{PPC}	0.01
Upper intestine lumen ↔ tissue	K_{PUI}	0.01
Lower intestine lumen ↔ tissue	K_{PLI}	0.01

to chemical uptake from the diet. The shape of this line parallels that given for growth dilution, but the actual shape will depend on the relationship between dietary assimilation efficiency and log KOW. Across a range of log KOW values the extent of biomagnification is determined by the balance between dietary uptake and branchial efflux. Branchial efflux is unlikely to important, however, at log KOW values greater than 7. All of these relationships provide the backdrop for a fourth line (dot-dash) which shows the possible impact of metabolic biotransformation. To date, PBTK models for fish have not been used in ecological risk assessment. The mechanistic perspective required for model development has contributed substantially, however, to our current understanding of chemical kinetics in fish, indirectly improving such assessments. In time, it is hoped that research on high log KOW compounds will yield the information needed to transform hypothetical relationships shown in Figure 13 into validated model predictions.

6.8 References

Abbas R, and Hayton WL. 1997. A physiologically based pharmacokinetic and pharmacodynamic model for paraoxon in rainbow trout. Toxicol. Appl. Pharmacol. 145:192-201.

Andersen ME, Mills JJ, Gargas ML, Kedderis L, Birnbaum LS, Neubert D, and Greenlee WF. 1993. Modeling receptor-mediated processes with dioxin: implications for pharmacokinetics and risk assessment. Risk Anal. 13:25-36.

Barber MC, Suarez LS, and Lassiter RR. 1991. Modelling bioaccumulation of organic pollutants in fish with an application to PCBs in Lake Ontario Salmonids. Can. J. Fish. Aquat. Sci. 48:318-337.

Bergman A, Brandt I, Darnerud PO, and Wachtmeister CA. 1982. Metabolism of 2,2',5,5'-tetrachlorobiphenyl: formation of mono- and bis-methyl sulphone metabolites with a selective affinity for the lung and kidney tissues in mice. Xenobiotica 12:1-7.

Bergman A, Klasson-Wehler E, and Kuroki H. 1994. Selective retention of hydroxylated PCB metabolites in blood. Environ. Health Perspec. 102:464-469.

Bertelsen SL, Hoffman AD, Gallinat CA, Elonen CM, and Nichols JW. 1998. Evaluation of log Kow and tissue lipid content as predictors of chemical partitioning to fish tissues. Environ. Toxicol. Chem. 17:1447-1455.

Bruggeman WA, Opperhuizen A, Wijbenga A, and Hutzinger O. 1984. Bioaccumulation of super-lipophilic chemicals in fish. Toxicol. Environ. Chem. 7:173-189.

Bungay PM, Dedrick RL, Guarino AM. 1976. Pharmacokinetic modeling of the dogfish shark (Squalus acanthias): Distribution and urinary and biliary excretion of phenol red and its glucuronide. J. Pharmacokin. Biopharm. 4:377-388.

Bungay PM, Dedrick RL, Matthews HB. 1980. Enteric transport of chlordecone (Kepone®) in the rat. J. Pharmacokinet. Biopharm. 9:309-341.

Burreau S, Axelman J, Broman D, and Jakobsson E. 1997. Dietary uptake in pike (Esox lucius) of some polychlorinated biphenyls, polychlorinated naphthalenes and polybrominated diphenyl ethers administered in natural diet. Environ. Toxicol. Chem. 16:2508-2513.

Connolly JP, and Pedersen CJ. 1988. A thermodynamic-based evaluation of organic chemical accumulation in aquatic organisms. Environ. Sci. Technol. 22:99-103.

DeJongh J, Verhaar HJM, and Hermens JLM. 1997. A quantitative property-property relationship (QPPR) approach to estimate in vitro tissue-blood partition coefficients of organic chemicals in rats and humans. Arch. Toxicol. 72:17-25.

Erickson RJ, and McKim JM. 1990a. A simple flow-limited model for exchange of organic chemicals at fish gills. Environ. Toxicol. Chem. 9:159-165.

Erickson RJ, and McKim JM. 1990b. A model for exchange of organic chemicals at fish gills: flow and diffusion limitations. Aquat. Toxicol. 18:175-198.

Fitzsimmons PN, Fernandez JD, Hoffman AD, Butterworth BC, and Nichols JW. 2001. Branchial elimination of hydrophobic organic compounds by rainbow trout (Oncorhynchus mykiss). Aquat. Toxicol. (in press).

Gargas ML, Burgess RJ, Voisard DE, Cason GH, and Andersen ME. 1989. Partition coefficients of low molecular weight volatile chemicals in various liquids and tissues. Toxicol. Appl. Pharmacol. 98:87-99.

Gobas FAPC, Muir DCG, Mackay D. 1988. Dynamics of dietary bioaccumulation and faecal elimination of hydrophobic organic chemicals in fish. Chemosphere17:943-962.

Gobas FAPC, Zhang X, Wells R. 1993. Gastrointestinal magnification: The mechanism of biomagnification and food chain accumulation of organic chemicals. Environ. Sci. Technol. 27:2855-2863.

Gobas FAPC, Wilcockson JB, Russell RW, and Haffner GD. 1999. Mechanism of biomagnification in fish under laboratory and field conditions. Environ. Sci. Technol. 33:133-141.

Hoffman AD, Bertelsen SL, and Gargas ML. 1992. An in vitro gas equilibration method for determination of chemical partition coefficients in fish. Comp. Biochem. Physiol. 101:47-51.

Jepson GW, Hoover DK, Black RK, McCafferty JD, Mahle DA, and Gearhart JM. 1994. A partition coefficient determination method for nonvolatile chemicals in biological tissues. Fund. Appl. Toxicol. 22:519-524.

Johnson RD, Tietge JE, Jensen KM, Fernandez JD, Lothenbach DL, Holcombe GW, Cook PM, Drummond R, Christ S, Lattier D, Gordon D. 1998. Toxicity of 2,3,7,8-TCDD to F1 generation brook trout (Salvelinus fontinalis) exposed via parental generation. Environ. Toxicol. Chem. 17:2408-2421.

Kedderis LB, Mills JJ, Andersen ME, and Birnbaum LS. 1993. A physiologically based pharmacokinetic model for 2,3,7,8-tetrabromodibenzo-p-dioxin (TBDD) in the rat: tissue distribution and CYP1A induction. Toxicol Appl. Pharmacol. 121:87-98.

Law FCP, Abenini S, and Kennedy CJ. 1991. A biologically based toxicokinetic model for pyrene in rainbow trout. Toxicol. Appl. Pharmacol. 110:390-402.

Mackay D. 1982. Correlation of bioconcentration factors. Environ. Sci. Technol. 16:274-278.

McCarthy JF, and Jimenez BD. 1985. Interactions between polycyclic aromatic hydrocarbons and dissolved humic material: binding and dissociation. Environ. Sci. Technol. 19:1072-1076.

McKim JM, and Nichols JW. 1994. The use of physiologically-based models in a mechanistic approach to aquatic toxicology. In Malins DC, Ostrander GK, eds, Aquatic Toxicology: Molecular, Biochemical, and Cellular Perspectives. Lewis, Boca Raton, FL, USA, pp 469-519.

Miller MA. 1993. Maternal transfer of organochlorine compounds in salmonines to their eggs. Can. J. Fish. Aquat. Sci. 50:1405-1413.

Murphy JE, Janszen DB, and Gargas ML. 1995. An in vitro method for determination of tissue partition coefficients of non-volatile chemicals such as 2,3,7,8- tetrachlorodibenzo-p-dioxin and estradiol. J. Appl. Toxicol. 15:147-152.

Nichols JW. 1999. Recent advances in the development and use of physiologically based toxicokinetic models for fish. In: Xenobiotics in Fish. D.J. Smith, W. Gingerich, and M.Beconi-Baker, Eds., Plenum, New York, pp. 87-104.

Nichols JW, McKim JM, Andersen ME, Gargas ML, Clewell HJ III, Erickson RJ. 1990. A physiologically based toxicokinetic model for the uptake and disposition of waterborne organic chemicals in fish. Toxicol Appl Pharm 106:433-447.

Nichols JW, McKim JM, Lien GJ, Hoffman AD, and Bertelsen SH. 1991. Physiologically based toxicokinetic modeling of three chlorinated ethanes in rainbow trout (Oncorhynchus mykiss). Toxicol. Appl. Pharm. 110:374-389.

Nichols JW, McKim JM, Lien GJ, Hoffman AD, Bertelsen SL, and Elonen CM. 1996. A physiologically-based toxicokinetic model for dermal absorption of organic chemicals by fish. Fund. Appl. Toxicol. 31:229-242.

Nichols JW, Jensen KM, Tietge JE, and Johnson RD. 1998. A physiologically based toxicokinetic model for maternal transfer of 2,3,7,8-tetrachlorodibenzo-p-dioxin in brook trout (Salvelinus fontinalis). Environ. Toxicol. Chem. 17:2422-2434.

Nichols JW, Fitzsimmons PN, Whiteman FW, Kuehl DW, Butterworth BC, and Jenson CT. 2001. Dietary uptake kinetics of 2,2',5,5'-tetrachlorobiphenyl in rainbow trout. Drug Metab. Disposit. (in press).

Poland A, Teitelbaum P, and Glover E. 1989. [125]2-Iodo-3,7,8-trichlorodibenzo-p- dioxin-binding species in mouse liver induced by agonists for the Ah receptor: Characterization and identification. Mol. Pharmacol. 36:113-120.

Poulin P, Krishnan K. 1995. An algorithm for predicting tissue:blood partition coefficients of organic chemicals from n-octanol:water partition coefficient data. J. Toxicol. Environ. Health 46:117-129.

Poulin P, Krishnan K. 1996. A tissue composition-based algorithm for predicting tissue:air partition coefficients of organic chemicals. Toxicol. Appl. Pharmacol. 136:126-130.

Russell RW, Gobas FAPC, and Haffner GD. 1999. Role of chemical and ecological factors in trophic transfer of organic chemicals in aquatic food webs. Environ. Toxicol. Chem. 18:1250-1257.

Tietge JE, Johnson RD, Jensen KM, Cook PM, Elonen GE, Fernandez JD, Holcombe GW, Lothenbach DL, Nichols JW. 1998. Reproductive toxicity and disposition of 2,3,7,8 tetrachlorodibenzo-p-dioxin in adult brook trout (Salvelinus fontinalis) following a dietary exposure. Environ. Toxicol. Chem. 17:2395-2407.

Zaharko DS, Dedrick RL, and Oliverio VT. 1972. Prediction of the distribution of methotrexate in the sting rays Dasyatidae sabina and sayi by use of a model developed in mice. Comp. Biochem. Physiol., 42:183-194.

7 CHAIR'S INTRODUCTION TO THE SECOND SYMPOSIUM DAY

PETER C. BRAGT

Senior Officer, Inspectorate for Health Protection, Commodities and Veterinary Public Health, Ministry of Health, Welfare and Sports, The Netherlands

7.1 Introduction

In 1997, the Netherlands Society of Toxicology organized a symposium chaired by Dr. Henk Derks of the National Institute of Public Health and the Environment (RIVM[1]) under the provocative title: "*PBPK models: where's the beef?*". The themes of this symposium were presented by excellent national speakers and an international keynote speaker. Guided by merely this title, one might perhaps draw the preliminary conclusion that PBPK models belong to mysticism and are made and used by mathematicians, just for their own satisfaction. One would also wonder whether there could be any benefit for society of such high degree academic constructs that are so little transparent for uninitiated people.

However, what became apparent during this symposium? There are no mystics anymore about PBPK models. These models can be made as transparent as desired. There have been revolutions in applied mathematics and computers during the last decade, and PBPK models have become available for a broad range of applications and a large number of scientists of different disciplines. The main conclusion of the symposium was that the beef is already being consumed, and ...with great appetite! There was also a serious warning signal. Models are abundantly available nowadays and can be used with low thresholds on personal computer systems. The models will produce results, even in the hands of absolute laymen. The obvious question is then: are the results obtained by a model meaningful? Are they reliable? An example was presented of a so-called "adjusted" liver compartment with a volume of 50 litres, which of course by far exceeds the pathophysiological size limits of hepatomegaly, even in the heaviest drinker of alcohol.

From many scientific papers as well as the titles and abstracts of this symposium it is clear that toxicokinetic models are indispensable nowadays.

J. Krüse, H.J.M. Verhaar, and W.K. de Raat (eds.), The Practical Applicability of Toxicokinetic Models in the Risk Assessment of Chemicals, 135-139.

From my personal experience, not as a scientist, but as a public health officer, I can endorse the merits of modelling for risk assessment in the field of consumer protection against hazardous chemicals, both for regulation and enforcement purposes. In 1991, initial attempts were made by RIVM to start a modelling program, and the Inspectorate for Health Protection was asked to sponsor this program with capacity input from the available capacity pool of about 70 man-years. Within two years the modelling activities appeared so successful that the RIVM management decided to cluster these activities in a cluster called "modelling and development methods for risk assessment". Ever since, many reports that contained modelling as an essential part of the quantitative risk assessment have been published by RIVM.

Let me briefly guide you through some practical examples of modelling, that were used in The Netherlands for regulation or enforcement activities in the field of public health protection.

7.2 Cancer risk assessment of azo dyes and aromatic amines from garment and footwear (Speijers et al, 1996; Zeilmaker et al. 1999).

Our government wanted insight in the cancer risk of azo dyes and their decomposition products, the aromatic amines, to decide whether legislation had to be made. Samples were obtained from the Dutch market and investigated on their azo dye release by the Inspectorate. Subsequently, RIVM developed a model that took into account

1. the chance that garments and footwear contain azo dyes,
2. the frequency of wearing
3. the fraction of the material that comes into contact with the skin
4. the concentration of aromatic amines
5. the migration of azo dyes and amines
6. skin absorption of azo dyes and amines
7. the USEPA dose-response slope for bladder cancer as the critical endpoint of benzidine exposure.

From the risk assessment based on the modelling, it became apparent that the cancer risk under reasonable worst-case conditions is much higher than the negligible risk level (one extra tumour per 10^6 people exposed for lifetime). For some textile samples, even the maximal permissible risk level (10^{-4}) was exceeded. As a consequence, the Minister of Health established a regulation on azo dyes within the framework of the Food and Commodities Act (Warenwet).

7.3 Calculation of human toxicity thresholds for TCDD (Zeilmaker and Van Eijkeren, 1998)

To answer the question which no-effect levels exist for the toxicity of dioxins to different organ systems in man, a model was developed by RIVM. The model included:

1. variability and uncertainty of TCDD kinetics
2. variation in terminal dioxin half-life
3. tenfold higher sensitivity of man to TCDD effects than rat, equal sensitivity monkey and man
4. presence or absence of extrahepatic protein binding of dioxin

Using the model, the following no-effect levels for TCDD were calculated:
<u>hepatotoxicity:</u> an intake of34 and 54 pg/kg.d with and without extra-hepatic protein binding
<u>cardiovascular and pulmonary toxicity:</u> 2 and 3 pg/kg.d
<u>embryotoxicity:</u> 8 and 10 pg/kg.d
<u>endometriosis in women:</u> 5 pg/kg.d (model without extrahepatic protein binding)
<u>disturbed cognitive development in offspring from exposed mothers:</u>
3 pg/kg.d (model without extrahepatic protein binding).

7.4 PBPK simulated adduct formation as a result of benzopyrene administration (Zeilmaker et al, 1997-1999).

The model takes into account:

1. uptake, distribution, metabolism of B[a]P
2. DNA adduct formation in the liver
3. induction of B[a]P metabolizing enzymes (CYP 1A1 and CYP 1A2)
4. adduct accumulation in the liver

With the model, the effects of single or repetitive oral and intravenous administration on the formation of DNA adducts in the target organ for carcinogenesis, the liver, can be studied. A virtually safe dose (VSD) for B[a]P in the range of 1.3-27 ng/kg.d was calculated from the simulated DNA adduct formation.

When based on the administered B[a]P dose, the VSD was calculated to be 57 ng/kg.d. From these modelling activities, It is clear that further refinement of risk assessment is feasible if mechanistic data are taken into consideration. It must be stressed here, that the opportunities for these modelling activities were greatly facilitated by the in-house chronic oral carcinogenesis bio-assay in rats at the request of the Inspectorate for Health Protection, with the aim to arrive at a VSD for B[a]P and poly-aromatic hydrocarbons (PAH) in the diet.

7.5 Model for estimating lipophilic contaminants in cattle (Freijer et al, 1999).

One aspect of the European food legislation is the high level of protection against contaminants in the food. Among the sources of contaminants in our diet are the milk and meat from cattle. RIVM developed a model for the assessment of historical exposures of cattle on basis of measured contaminant levels in milk and meat samples obtained by my veterinary colleagues.

The model was, I would say, a classical PBPK model. However, it is used in a very creative way. Namely, instead of predicting tissue concentrations from administered dose levels, the model does in fact the opposite. The model is intended for use as a screening tool by veterinary inspectors in order to have an impression of exposures, residues and the health risks associated herewith. The model has been validated by introducing TCDD into the rumen of lactating and non-lactating cows and lindane, and certain PCB congeners to lactating and non-lactating goats.

7.6 Last, but certainly not at least, the modelling of consumer exposure (Van Veen et al, 1994-now).

Much attention has been paid to modelling in the toxicology. Up to the mid of the nineties, toxicologists were able to provide risk managers with refined risk assessments, based on excellent toxicological data and elegant mathematical models to predict the detailed kinetics of a substance and its target organ concentration. However, in most instances the exposure parameters were not more than just "guesstimates". In view of the paradigm that the risk of people is determined by both hazard and exposure, the reliability of the ultimate risk figure is very low, when the exposure predictions are bad. Therefore, at the request of the Ministry of Health, RIVM has invested a lot in the building of an appropriate generic model for the exposure of consumers to chemical substances. This model is the so-called Consexpo model. Briefly, on basis of contact scenario's, exposure scenario's and uptake scenario's, the model is able to define a stochastically distributed dose parameter, which can be compared with known toxicological threshold values. Much effort is paid to the acquisition of data, either from literature or from validation experiments, to describe the aforementioned scenarios for consumer products appropriately.

Personally, I expect much benefit of this exposure model to be applied on behalf of an activity of CEN Technical Committee 52 Workgroup 9, on the chemical safety of toys. You should imagine that about 800 (!) organic-chemical substances have been annotated as priority chemicals recently. These substances may occur in a variety of toys, from baby teethers, finger paints, crayons and face masks to playtents, each toy category with its own contact and exposure characteristics, and each substance with its own physicochemical properties. I am sure that exposure modelling will be of much help to set standards for these great many organochemicals.

Back to the present day of the symposium, now. Modelling of the sequence

exposure → dose at contact site with body → delivered dose → target organ concentration → adverse effect

with relevance for human health risk assessment is the central theme of this symposium.

Today's session focuses mainly on:

1. The relevance of what happens in the target organ, either at a local or a systemic site. Dr. Annette Kopp-Schneider will present an overview of statistic versus mechanistic models of carcinogenesis with their potentials and limitations. Dr. Annie Jarabek will bring the mode of action into your attention and the relevance of toxicological data and principles for risk managers, among which the regulators. She will also present examples of chemical substances that display specific modes of action. At the end of the day, Dr. Bas Blaauboer will demonstrate the power of utilization and combination of existing data to predict local and systemic toxic effects of chemical substances.
2. The choice of the right PBPK model on behalf of the regulatory process. Dr. Sean Hays will discuss the use of PBPK models to understand the mechanisms of toxicity, e.g. neurotoxicity and carcinogenicity. He will focus on a number of different chemicals.
3. Finally, a summary and conclusions about the current state of the art by the organizers of this symposium, represented by Dr. Karel de Raat.

I am confident that the outcome of this symposium will be of much benefit to the participants that either build PBPK models themselves, or that are users, or should I say "*consumers*", of such model for decision making in private companies or in the government as part of the regulatory process.

8 CAN BIOLOGICALLY BASED MODELS OF CARCINOGENESIS BE USED FOR RISK ASSESSMENT ?

Potentials and limitations of carcinogenesis models

ANNETTE KOPP-SCHNEIDER

Senior Statistician, Central Unit Biostatistics, German Cancer Research Center, Heidelberg, Germany.

Summary: In their 1996 proposed guidelines, the United States Environmental Protection Agency (US EPA 1996) suggest the use of biologically based carcinogenesis models for low-dose risk estimation in cancer risk assessment whenever sufficient data are available in support of the model. In this contribution, an overview of carcinogenesis models is presented and the models are classified according to their ability to incorporate biological detail. The utility of these models for risk assessment is discussed and two different applications are distinguished: either the models can be used for low-dose extrapolation or for risk prediction. In the first application, one has to cope with two challenges: to carefully select the model for correct representation of the mechanism and to then choose the appropriate dose-response relationship for each model parameter. As an example of risk prediction, the model can be used to analyze scenarios for different dose-response relationships of the model parameters and their impact on the shape of lifetime tumor probability.

8.1 Introduction

It is a well-recognized paradigm in cancer research that "Carcinogenesis involves progression from a normal to an initiated state and then to an overtly malignant state. It is associated with the development of multiple genetic and/or epigenetic defects in oncogenes and/or cancer suppressor genes" (R. E. Scott et al. 1993). A number of genetic and epigenetic alterations have been identified that are associated with carcinogenesis. Cancer might be enhanced by the action of chemicals through changes in mutational events, cell proliferation behavior or cell death.

Risk assessment deals with the evaluation of the toxic or carcinogenic properties of a chemical substance and the conditions of human exposure. The assessment usually consists of four steps: hazard identification, dose-response assessment, exposure assessment and risk characterization (US EPA 1995). In carcinogenesis risk assessment, the endpoint of interest is the occurrence of a malignant tumor in lifetime. The main goal in risk assessment is to find a dose corresponding to an 'acceptable cancer risk' caused by

J. Krüse, H.J.M. Verhaar, and W.K. de Raat (eds.), The Practical Applicability of Toxicokinetic Models in the Risk Assessment of Chemicals, 141-153.

the substance. Often the acceptable excess risk is chosen to be of the order 10^{-6} and the corresponding dose is then perceived as 'virtually safe'.

Although the ultimate goal obviously is to assess risk in humans, the main tool for estimating a virtually safe dose is to derive a low dose estimate for the most sensitive animal species and to then transfer this estimate to the human situation. This dose estimate however cannot be determined experimentally. Animal studies usually include 50 animals per dose group, hence 2% is the smallest increase compared to background which can be observed. Therefore, low dose risk estimation needs to rely on the quantification of the dose-response relationship for lifetime tumor risk. Usually, a functional relationship describing tumor probability in dependence of dose and time is called a carcinogenesis model.

One important issue in cancer risk assessment is the shape of the dose-response function in the low-dose region. Specifically, risk regulators want to know if the carcinogenesis model predicts a low-dose linear behavior, a term used for the situation that the slope of the dose-response curve is greater than zero for dose=0. If the slope of the dose-response curve is zero for dose=0, then a small increase in dose will result in virtually no change in the tumor prevalence. However, if the slope is greater zero, the change in tumor prevalence will be proportional to dose. Hence dose-response functions that are low-dose linear yield smaller estimates of acceptable exposure than dose-response functions that are not low-dose linear.

8.2 Models of carcinogenesis

A number of models have been suggested to describe the process of carcinogenesis. They all describe the tumor probability as a function of time, dose of the substance and some additional parameters. Generally, these models are applied to interpolate (estimation of TD50) or extrapolate in dose (estimation of the virtually safe dose), to quantify the carcinogenicity of a substance in order to compare the carcinogenicity of different substances and, in epidemiology, to compare cancer incidence in different populations.

The models that have been suggested in the past 50 years can be classified according to their intention, to the biological detail they include and to the methodological approach that is used for the analysis as shown in Fig. 1.

The most commonly known models are the statistical models. The log-probit model assumes that each individual has a tolerance for the carcinogenic agent and that these tolerance limits follow a lognormal distribution. The most frequently used statistical model for carcinogenesis is the Weibull-model:

$$P(T \leq t) = 1 - e^{-\sigma t^{\kappa}} \text{ with } \sigma, \kappa > 0,$$

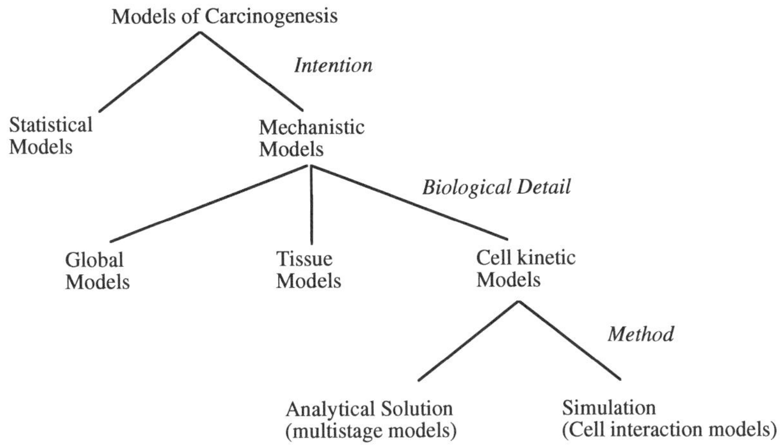

Figure 1. A classification of stochastic models of carcinogenesis.

where T denotes the time to tumor. The Weibull distribution is used as a lifetime distribution in reliability theory because it describes the failure of a system of independent components where all components are necessary for the function of the system. These statistical models have some mechanistic justification, estimated parameters of the models however cannot be interpreted in a biological framework.

Mechanistic models instead have been suggested and applied because they incorporate biological hypotheses and have biologically interpretable parameters that can be measured directly or compared to experimental results. They therefore represent a powerful tool for testing biological hypotheses and to draw inference about the process of carcinogenesis. The risk assessment community has placed some hope into the usefulness of these mechanistic models for reliable estimates in the low dose range.

Mechanistic models exist for different levels of biological detail: they may be formulated to describe the process of cancer formation on the level of the organism or on the level of tissues which go through irreversible changes to host a malignant tumor. Most models are formulated at the cellular level. The long range goal however will certainly be to describe carcinogenesis even on the lower level of intracellular events such as DNA-adducts and gene expression. However, it should be kept in mind that a model can only be called mechanistic if it uses the information on the level it is designed for. If a cell kinetic model is used to describe time to tumor data without any information about premalignant cell populations and without information on the cellular level such as rates of cell division or cell death, then it is used as a purely statistical model, providing only a formula for the tumor incidence function.

The most prominent biologically based models, often called multistage models, are formulated at the cellular level, describing the malignant transformation of normal cells as a process involving mutations, cell proliferation/differentiation and occasionally repair. They commonly assume that a cell has to go through k (> 1) mutational changes and that intermediate cells are subject to a birth/death process. The basic assumption for all of these models is that cells act independently, i.e. that a tissue is nothing more than the sum of its cells. This unrealistic assumption is necessary to treat them in the framework of stochastic processes, hence allowing for explicit analytic expressions for the parameters of interest or at least for fast numerical algorithms to calculate these parameters. More realistic incorporating cell to cell interaction cannot be solved analytically and can only be investigated by computer simulation methods, making it virtually impossible to estimate model parameters by rigorous statistical techniques.

In all multistage models, it is assumed that the time from first malignant cell to overt carcinoma is very short compared to the time which is needed for a malignant cell to be generated and hence the time to carcinoma is very often approximated by the time to first malignant cell. In other cases, the time from first malignant cell to the detectable carcinoma may be assumed constant but fixed. This only calls for a transformation of the data to derive the time of the formation of the first malignant from the time of tumor diagnosis.

The Armitage-Doll model

Armitage and Doll (1954, 1957) suggested that a malignant cell is generated by a sequence of k irreversible changes and they investigated the quantitative implications of this approach. This concept - called multistage theory then - found widespread application since it combined biological plausibility with applicability to data sets from experimental and epidemiological studies. It is schematically shown in Figure 2.

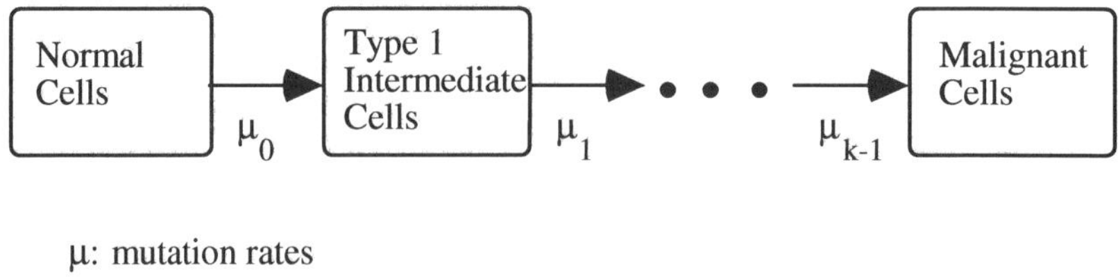

Figure 2. The Armitage-Doll model.

The distribution of the time to first malignant cell in the Armitage-Doll multistage model depicted in Figure 2 can be approximated by (Whittemore & Keller 1978)

$$P(T \leq t) \approx 1 - \exp\left\{ -\frac{x_0 \mu_0 \cdots \mu_{k-1}}{k!} t^k \right\}$$

Kendall (1960) proposed a model with a subcritical birth-death process for intermediate and a supercritical birth-death process for malignant cells. Moolgavkar and Venzon (1979) formulated a two-stage model with stochastic clonal expansion of both normal and intermediate cells and they introduced a mathematical technique to analyze a two-stage model with deterministic growth of normal cells and stochastic growth of intermediate cells. Moolgavkar and Knudson (1981) discussed the application of this model to epidemiological and experimental data. Although originally this model was proposed by Kendall, it is often termed the MVK model. The model with stochastic growth of normal and intermediate cells is depicted in Figure 3.

The model can be used to describe both premalignant and malignant lesions. It accounts for phenomena observed in initiation/promotion studies: an initiating agent produces a number of lesions which are expanded through the action of a promoting substance.

Again, the time to overt tumor is here approximated by the time to first malignant cell. It has been common to use an approximation suggested by Whittemore and Keller (1978) to describe the time to tumor. However, various studies have shown that this approximation is inexact (e.g. Moolgavkar et al. 1988, Kopp & Portier 1989), especially in situations where tumor probability is high. These situations can be characterized as those where the second mutation rate $\mu_I\beta_I$ is high or where net proliferation of intermediate

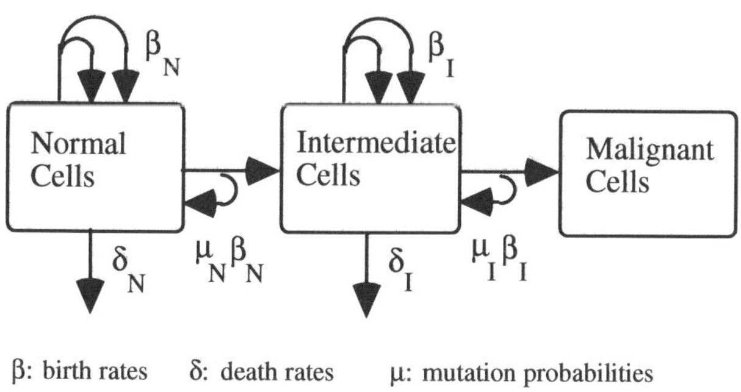

Figure 3. The two-stage model with clonal expansion

cells β_I - δ_I is large. They occur most commonly in experimental carcinogenesis studies.

More recently, the exact solution for the distribution function of tumor onset has been derived for time constant rates (Kopp-Schneider et al. 1994, Zheng 1994):

$$P(T \le t) =$$
$$= 1 - \exp\left\{ -\frac{x_0 \mu_N \beta_N}{\beta_I} \left[t \frac{\beta_I - \delta_I - \mu_I \beta_I + r}{2} + \ln\left(\frac{\delta_I - \beta_I + \mu_I \beta_I + r + (\beta_I - \delta_I - \mu_I \beta_I + r) e^{-rt}}{2r} \right) \right] \right\}$$

where $r = \sqrt{[\beta_I + \delta_I + \mu_I \beta_I]^2 - 4\beta_I \delta_I}$.

This equation is not essentially more complicated than the approximate solution and therefore it is strongly recommended to use it whenever the distribution function for the time to first malignant cell has to be calculated.

Another method for numerical calculation of the distribution function of tumor onset is the solution of a system of differential equations which is derived from the Kolmogorov backwards equations (e.g. Portier et al. 1996). This algorithm even produces solutions when the birth, death and mutation rates are non-constant functions of time.

It should be noted however, that the 4 model parameters carcinogenesis $x_0\mu_N\beta_N$, β_I, δ_I and μ_I are not identifiable when estimated from tumor data only (Heidenreich 1996). For a unique solution of these 4 parameters, information about premalignant cells is necessary. Otherwise, only 3 of the 4 parameters can be estimated.

The theory of stochastic processes - especially the theory of filtered Poisson processes together with the theory of birth-death processes - can be used to derive the number and size distribution of intermediate cell clones. It is possible to derive these distributions for piecewise constant mutation rates and with a piecewise constant ratio of death to birthrate (Kopp-Schneider 1992).

The two-stage model with clonal expansion has been applied to epidemiological time to tumor-data, e.g. for carcinoma of the breast (Moolgavkar et al. 1980), colon (Moolgavkar et al. 1992) and lung (Moolgavkar et al. 1993) as well as lymphocytic leukemia (Little et al. 1996). It has been used for experimental lung cancer data (Moolgavkar, Cross et al. 1990). Since it can be used to describe the premalignant stage, it has been applied to experimental data on premalignant clones such as mouse skin papillomas (Kopp-Schneider and Portier 1992), mouse skin papillomas and carcinomas (Kopp-Schneider and Portier 1995) and liver foci (e.g. Moolgavkar, Luebeck et al. 1990, Moolgavkar et al. 1996, Portier et al. 1996). In all these situations, application of the model was performed by Maximum Likelihood estimation, i.e. by formulating the likelihood of the data and maximizing this likelihood with respect to the model parameters.

It should be stressed that application of this type of mechanistic model involves derivation of the quantities of interest in the framework of stochastic processes and the translation of the resulting equations into computer code to calculate the Maximum-Likelihood estimates for the parameters, tasks that exceed standard statistical techniques.

8.3 Quantitative risk assessment with multistage models

The application of carcinogenesis models for cancer risk assessment requires that dose is incorporated into these models. Different possibilities exist in which dose of a putative carcinogenic substance can enter into a model, the model parameters depending on dose either in an additive or an independent manner (Portier 1987). In this context, an additive effect indicates that exposure to the substance under study augments an ongoing process. This may be realized by expressing the model parameters, i.e. the birth, death, mutation and repair rates, as a function of dose. An independent effect of exposure on the other hand refers to a situation in which the substance under study causes a new mechanism of malignant transformation. This may be described by a two-pathway model, one pathway reflecting the generation of spontaneous tumors whereas the other pathway represents the mechanism of carcinogenesis caused by the agent. Since most research has addressed additive instead of independent effects of dose on one or several parameters of the models, this is what will be discussed in the present manuscript.

Models of carcinogenesis can be used for two tasks in risk assessment. The most important challenge for risk assessment is the estimation of risk in the low dose region. However, another challenge is risk prediction, i.e. the description of the relationship between dose and time to tumor if specified dose-response relationships hold for the model parameters.

The United States Environmental Protection Agency has a long history of using multistage models for low dose risk estimation. In their currently valid guidelines of 1986 (US EPA 1986), they suggest the use of the linearized version of the Armitage-Doll model, the so-called 'linearized multistage model' as a default method for cancer risk assessment. In their more recently proposed new guidelines for risk assessment (US EPA 1996) the EPA draws back from the use of the linearized multistage model as a default with the argument that using the linearized multistage model 'gave an appearance of specific knowledge and sophistication unwarranted for a default' (US EPA 1996). Instead, they now propose to use a biologically based or case specific model whenever data are available to support the model. Inherent in this new policy concerning low-dose extrapolation is the belief that use of a biologically based model will yield better estimates in the low-dose range.

Two challenges are connected with the application of the new guidelines. First, the risk assessor must choose the appropriate mechanistic model for application to the data. Different models that might be applied will be discussed later as well as the question of model adequacy for known models. Once the mechanism of carcinogenesis is translated into the model, the second problem is the incorporation of dose into the model parameters. Several dose-response relationships for the dose-dependency of the parameters may be used and the choice of the correct one is crucial for the full model to be applicable for risk assessment.

The second application of mechanistic models for risk assessment is risk prediction through the analysis of hypothetic situations: suppose a mechanistic model is valid and assume dose-response relationships for the model parameters, one can investigate dose-effects on the variables of interest such as the distribution function of tumor onset.

Quantitative risk assessment with the Armitage-Doll model

Dose effects in the Armitage-Doll model have been studied and used extensively. Incorporating dose into the distribution function for time to first malignant cell in the Armitage-Doll model by assuming that the mutation rates, μ_i, are linear functions of dose d, i.e. $\mu_i(d) = a_i + b_i d$ the probability of a tumor at a given time t can be expressed as

$$P(T(d) \le t) = 1 - \exp\left\{ -\sum_{i=0}^{k} q_i d^i \right\}$$

where the qi are derived from the number of normal cells x0, the time tk and the coefficients a_i and b_i. For small d,

$$\frac{P(T(d) \le t) - P(T(0) \le t)}{1 - P(T(0) \le t)} \approx q_1 d \, .$$

Hence q_1 represents the slope of the dose-response curve in the low-dose region, showing that the Armitage-Doll model is low-dose linear. The EPA advocated the use of the upper 95% confidence limit, q_1*, for risk assessment.

The Armitage-Doll model has been used to draw inferences concerning the mechanism of action of carcinogenic substances (Whittemore 1977, Day and Brown 1980). Exposure to a single carcinogen leads to different patterns of age-specific cancer incidence rates depending upon the stage affected by the carcinogen. When the carcinogen affects only the first stage of the process, the excess incidence depends on exposure duration and continues to rise after exposure ends, whereas a carcinogen affecting only the penultimate stage leads to excess incidence that remains fixed at the level attained at the end of exposure. In situations of joint exposure to two carcinogens, an additive relative risk relationship is observed when the carcinogens affect the same stage of the process.

Quantitative risk assessment with the two-stage model with clonal expansion

If biologically based models are used for risk estimation in the low dose range as mechanistic and not only as statistical models, some knowledge about the cell kinetic parameters has to be available. Two approaches can be used for estimation of the dose-response relationship of the model parameters, a parametric one relying on a known functional form for the relationship between dose and model parameters and a non-parametric one independent of this knowledge (Kopp-Schneider 1997).

One can assume a dose-response relationship for each parameter of the model, as in the 'linearized multistage model', and then estimate the coefficients for these dose-response relationships, using them for the extrapolation to the low-dose range. This procedure looks as if a biologically based model was used for risk assessment, but unless the dose-response relationship for the model parameters can be derived by scientific arguments, it represents a sophisticated version of a statistical curve-fitting procedure. One way to justify parametric dose-response relationships for the model parameters would be to obtain them from a pharmacokinetic model, and this may be the best parametric approach for low-dose extrapolation.

Another approach to the use of multistage models for low-dose extrapolation consists of their application to combined data on tumor occurrence and cell kinetic parameters in a dose range where tumors can be observed. Thus, we can identify the model parameters that are affected by the substance under study, as well as estimate the dose independent parameters. Low-dose extrapolation would then be carried out by directly measuring the dose-dependent parameters in the low-dose region and use those in the appropriate model.

This, however, raises problems concerning the accuracy with which cell kinetic parameters can be measured, because multistage models are very sensitive to alterations in the cell kinetic parameters, especially for changes concerning the ratio of death to birth rates or the difference between those rates (Crump 1994a, 1994b). It would hardly be conceivable that estimates of the cell kinetic parameters - even if they were available - are accurate enough for use in risk assessment. For the estimation of cell kinetic parameters it is necessary to correctly identify the population of cells which are of interest for modeling purposes. If cell kinetic parameters of the intermediate cells in the two-stage models are to be estimated, it may be extremely difficult to identify the corresponding population of premalignant cells which have acquired one specific mutation and can go on to malignancy. Usually, only one of the kinetic parameters is directly estimated from an experiment; the others being estimated from the application of the two-stage model to benign or malignant tumor data. From this information an assessment is made as to whether the model does or does not succeed in describing the data.

It should be noted that the validity of risk assessment based upon models crucially depends on the choice of the appropriate mechanistic model, not only of the right dose-response model for the model parameters but also of the model itself, e.g. the number of stages necessary for malignant transformation. There are situations where the two-stage model is inappropriate. Kopp-Schneider and Portier (1995) used the two-stage model with clonal expansion to describe data about premalignant and malignant lesions from a mouse skin painting study using DMBA as initiator and TPA as promoter. The experiment consisted of 4 experimental groups distinguished by different durations of promoting treatment. It could be shown that the two-stage model was not able to fit the papilloma and carcinoma data simultaneously. A large variety of related models was applied to the data but nevertheless none of them could explain the data, not even one which assumed that a proportion of the papillomas are terminally benign and therefore do not consist of intermediate cells in terms of the model.

Using the two-stage model with clonal expansion of intermediate cells for risk prediction, the potential effects on the parameters of the models have been used to classify substances (Thorslund et al 1987). In short, initiators are substances increasing the first mutation rate μ_N whereas substances increasing the second mutation rate μ_I have been called completers. Promoters increase the clonal expansion of intermediate cells by altering their proliferation kinetics, β_I and/or δ_I. In addition, there may be substances which increase the number of cells susceptible for a first mutation. These have been called co-carcinogens. Finally, an agent may reduce the rate of transformation into malignant cells via different mechanisms and is then termed inhibitor. In practice, a substance involved in the carcinogenesis process will often have a combined effect on several parameters in the framework of the two-stage model and hence not be clearly classifiable into one of these 5 groups.

Research about the effect of additive and independent substance effects on shape of the dose-response function for the two-stage model with clonal expansion has been performed by Portier (1987). Kodell et al. (1991) investigated the effect of combined exposure to two carcinogens in the framework of the two-stage model by analytically discussing the resulting hazard functions, using the approximate formulation for the tumor incidence function.

The two-stage model has been used for the analysis of dose-response relationships assuming different functional forms for the mutation and cell turnover rates, taking the 2-year tumor probability in a typical rodent bioassay as the response to be modeled. Lutz and Kopp-Schneider (1999) specifically analyzed mutation rates linear in dose combined with J-shaped cell turnover rates. J-shaped cell turnover rates may be induced by induction of a cell-cycle delay through low-level DNA-damage and acceleration of the cell cycle at cytotoxic dose levels. Experimentally, a J-shaped dose-response for cell turnover rates has been observed in experiments with caffeic acid (Lutz et al. 1997). Combination of linear mutation rates with J-shaped cell turnover rates may lead to J-shaped curves for the dose-lifetime tumor probability relationship if dose dependency of the mutation rates is not too strong. This approach can be used for a quantitative estimation of threshold doses: the dose where lifetime tumor probability returns to the background level can be defined as a threshold in that specific situation.

8.4 Summary

There is an ongoing debate about the use of biologically based models for risk assessment. The primary use of these models is their ability to incorporate and test biological hypotheses about the mechanism of cancer formation and to suggest experiments to distinguish between different proposed mechanisms. In addition, some researchers have expressed their belief that these models can be used for more accurate estimates of risk in the low-dose region. One should however not rely upon a mechanistic model for estimation of an acceptable cancer risk without critically analyzing the appropriateness of the model for the given situation. Both the model itself, e.g. the number of stages, as well as the dose dependency of the model parameters have to be chosen adequately. For risk prediction however, these models are very well suited.

8.5 References

Armitage P, Doll R. (1954) The age distribution of cancer and a multi-stage theory of carcinogenesis. British Journal of Cancer 8: 1-12.

Armitage P, Doll R. (1957) A two-stage theory of carcinogenesis in relation to the age distribution of human cancer. British Journal of Cancer 11: 161-169.

Crump KS. (1994a) Limitations of biological models of carcinogenesis for low-dose extrapolation. Risk Analysis 14: 883-886.

Crump KS. (1994b) Use of mechanistic models to estimate low-dose cancer risks. Risk Analysis 14: 1033-1038.

Day NE, Brown CC. (1980) Multistage models and primary prevention of cancer. Journal of the National Cancer Institute 64: 977-989.

Heidenreich WF. (1996) On the parameters of the clonal expansion model. Radiat. Envir. Biophys. 35: 127-129.

Kendall DG. (1960) Birth-and-death processes, and the theory of carcinogenesis. Biometrika 47, 13-21.

Kodell RL, Krewski D, Zielinski JM. (1991) Additive and multiplicative relative risk in the two-stage clonal expansion model of carcinogenesis. Risk Analysis 11: 483-490.

Kopp A, Portier CJ. (1989) A note on approximating the cumulative distribution function of the time to tumor onset in multistage models. Biometrics 45: 1259-1263.

Kopp-Schneider A. (1992) Birth-death processes with piecewise constant rates. Statistics & Probability Letters 13: 121-127.

Kopp-Schneider A, Portier CJ. (1992) Birth and death/differentiation rates of papillomas in mouse skin. Carcinogenesis 13: 973-978.

Kopp-Schneider A, Portier CJ, Sherman CD. (1994) The exact formula for tumor incidence in the two-stage model. Risk Analysis 14: 1079-1080.

Kopp-Schneider A., Portier CJ. (1995) Carcinoma formation in NMRI mouse skin painting studies is a process suggesting greater than two stages. Carcinogenesis 16: 53-59.

Kopp-Schneider A. (1997) Carcinogenesis models for risk assessment. Statistical methods in Medical Research 6: 317-340.

Little MP, Muirhead CR, Stiller CA (1996) Modelling lymphocytic leukaemia incidence in England and Wales using generalizations of the two-mutation model of carcinogenesis of Moolgavkar, Venzon and Knudson. Statistics in Medicine 15:1003-1022.

Lutz W, Kopp-Schneider A. (1999) Threshold dose-response for tumor induction by genotoxic carcinogens modeled via cell-cycle delay. Toxicological Sciences 49: 110-115.

Lutz U, Lugli S, Bitsch A, Schlatter J, Lutz W (1997) Dose response for the stimulation of cell division by caffeic acid in forestomach and kidney of male F344 rat. Fundamental and Applied Toxicology 39: 131-137.

Moolgavkar SH, Venzon DJ. (1979) Two-event model for carcinogenesis: Incidence curves for childhood and adult tumors. Mathematical Biosciences 47: 55-77.

Moolgavkar SH, Day NE, Stevens RG (1980) Two-stage model for carcinogenesis: Epidemiology of breast cancer in females. Journal of the National Cancer Institute 65: 559-569.

Moolgavkar SH, Knudson AG. (1981) Mutation and cancer: A model for human carcinogenesis. Journal of the National Cancer Institute 66: 1037-1052.

Moolgavkar SH, Dewanji A, Venzon DJ. (1988) A stochastic two-stage model for cancer risk assessment. I. The hazard function and probability of tumor. Risk Analysis 8: 383-392.

Moolgavkar SH, Cross FT, Luebeck G, Deagle GE. (1990) A two-mutation model for radon-induced lung tumors in rats. Radiation Research 121: 28-37.

Moolgavkar SH, Luebeck EG, de Gunst M, Port RE, Schwarz M. (1990) Quantitative analysis of enzyme-altered foci in rat hepatocarcinogenesis experiments I: Single agent regimen. Carcinogenesis 11: 1271-1278.

Moolgavkar SH, Luebeck EG. (1992) Multistage carcinogenesis: Population-based model for colon cancer. Journal of the National Cancer Institute 84: 610-618.

Moolgavkar SH, Luebeck EG, Krewski D, Zielinski JM. (1993) Radon, cigarette smoke, and lung cancer: A reanalysis of the Colorado Plateau Uranium miner's data. American Journal of Epidemiology 4: 204-217.

Moolgavkar SH, Luebeck EG, Buchmann A, Bock KW. (1996) Quantitative analysis of enzyme-altered liver foci in rats initiated with Diethylnitrosamine and promoted with

2,3,7,8-Tetrachlorodibenzo-p-dioxin or 1,2,3,4,5,7,8-Heptachlorodibenzo-p-dioxin. Toxicology and Applied Pharmacology 138: 31-42.

Portier CJ. (1987) Statistical properties of a two-stage model of carcinogenesis. Environmental Health Perspectives 76: 125-131.

Portier CJ, Kopp-Schneider A, Sherman CD. (1996) Estimating tumor incidence rates in stochastic models of carcinogenesis. Mathematical Biosciences 135: 129-146.

Portier CJ, Sherman CD, Kohn M, Edler L, Kopp-Schneider A, Maronpot RM, Lucier G. (1996) Modeling the number and size of hepatic focal lesions following exposure to 2,3,7,8-TCDD. Toxicology and Applied Pharmacology 138: 20-30.

Scott RE, Wang, H, Tzen C-T. (1993) What is cancer? Can cancer be cured or prevented? In: New frontiers in cancer causation (Ed: Iversen OH). Taylor & Francis, Washington DC, USA. pp 29-44.

Thorslund TW, Brown CC, Charnley G. (1987) Biologically motivated cancer risk models. Risk Analysis 7: 109-119.

US Environmental Protection Agency (1986). Risk assessment guidelines of 1986. Washington DC: Office of Health and Environmental Assessment, EPA/600/8-87/045. United States Environmental Protection Agency. Washington DC, USA.

US Environmental Protection Agency (1995). The use of benchmark dose approach in health risk assessment. Risk assessment forum. United States Environmental Protection Agency. Washington DC, USA.

US Environmental Protection Agency (1996). Proposed Guidelines for Carcinogen Risk Assessment. Federal Register 61: 17960-18011.

Whittemore AS. (1977) The age distribution of human cancers for carcinogenic exposures of varying intensity. American Journal of Epidemiology 106: 418-432.

Whittemore AS, Keller JB. (1978) Quantitative theories of carcinogenesis. SIAM Review 20: 1-30.

Zheng Q. (1994) On the exact hazard and survival functions of the MVK stochastic carcinogenesis model. Risk Analysis 14: 1081-1084.

9 THE PREDICTION OF SYSTEMIC TOXICITY BY INTEGRATING THE RESULTS OF BIOKINETIC MODELS AND BIOLOGICALLY BASED *IN VITRO* TEST METHODS[a]

BAS J. BLAAUBOER[1]

[a] *This paper is based on the work for the ECITTS programme (1995-1998) and the ECVAM Task Force in Integrated Testing. The author wishes to acknowledge the contribution of the following people, who were involved in one or both activities: Joost DeJongh[1,8], Anna Forsby[2], J. Brian Houston[3], André Guillouzo[4], Martin D. Barratt[5], Marie Beckman[6] and Robert D. Combes[7]*

[1]*Research Institute of Toxicology, Utrecht University, Utrecht, The Netherlands;* [2]*Dept of Neurochemistry and Neurotoxicology, Stockholm University, Stockholm, Sweden;* [3] *Department of Pharmacy, University of Manchester, UK;* [4]*INSERM U456, Unité Detoxication et Réparation Tissulaire, Rennes, France;* [5]*Marlin Consultancy, Carlton, Bedford, UK;* [6] *National Board for Laboratory Animals (CFN), Stockholm, Sweden;* [7]*FRAME, Nottingham, UK,* [8]*Present address: Leiden Advanced Pharmacokinetics & Pharmacodynamics (LAP&P) Consultants.*

Summary: We have evaluated the possibilities to predict the systemic toxic doses of chemicals on the basis of an integration of data derived from *in vitro* biologically based test systems and physio-logically-based biokinetic modelling for a number of neurotoxic compounds. This study was part of the ERGATT/CFN Integrated Toxicity Testing Scheme (ECITTS). In this programme, biokinetic models were constructed, where possible solely on the basis of *in vitro*-derived parameters for biotransformation as well as on partition coefficients determined or calculated from physicochemical structures. A test battery for relevant neurotoxic endpoints was developed in one of the co-operating laboratories. Effective concentrations in the most relevant test formed the basis of a calculation of the compound's effective dose, making use of the biokinetic model. This formed the basis of the prediction of a compound's systemic toxicity for acute or (sub) chronic exposure, expressed as a Lower Observed Effect Level (LOEL). Both the kinetic and the dynamic models were compared with known *in vivo* data. In general, the predictions were in good agreement with these data. The discrepancy between estimated and experimental LOELs ranged from approximately a factor two, for compounds with a low toxicity (i.e. a high LOEL), to a factor 10, for compounds with a high toxicity (i.e. a low LOEL). Building on the experience gained in this programme a Task Force on Integrated Toxicity Testing has been established by the European Centre for the Validation of Alternative Methods (ECVAM). The Task Force proposed a generalised scheme for a step-wise (decision tree) procedure for the use of data derived from different approaches (structure, *in vitro* systems and computational models) in risk assessments. This scheme would allow for assessing risks of chemicals on the basis of non-animal studies or at least with a strongly reduced number of animals.

J. Krüse, H.J.M. Verhaar, and W.K. de Raat (eds.), The Practical Applicability of Toxicokinetic Models in the Risk Assessment of Chemicals, 155-171.

9.1 Introduction

Modern society is increasingly depending on the use of chemicals, e.g. as pharmaceuticals, personal care products, biocides, industrial products, compounds applied in the production of edible products, etc. The benefits of the application of these com-pounds or products should be in an appropriate balance with the possible risks associated with their use. Toxicological evaluations, mainly on the basis of animal experiments, presently form the basis of the assessment of these risks. Hazard identification and the assessment of levels for possible exposure(s) are the most prominent components of risk assessment [1]. The procedures for (animal-based) experiments are highly standardised, e.g. in the form of OECD guidelines, carried out under the rules of Good Laboratory Practice [2].

For the development of new chemical entities and products in industry, it is necessary to obtain information on their hazard at the appropriate time. Availability of data on unavoidable risks of the use of compounds will prevent the further development of a certain product containing this compound, which makes this knowledge of eminent economic value. This is especially true in a situation in which large numbers of chemicals are being produced (e.g. by combinatorial chemistry) and high-throughput systems can be applied for the identification of possible effective medicines. The selection of the most appropriate chemicals for further development can therefore only be made if data on possible risks will become available at an early stage in development. It will be clear that the standard procedures for a toxicological risk assessment based on animal experiments will not fulfil these requirements.

Risk assessment and its reliance on animal tests

The area of toxicological risk evaluation traditionally relies on a wide array of animal experiments, mostly in the form of standard procedures for which guidelines have been formulated by the OECD [2]. The day-to-day practice of these procedures has, in many cases, led to the relatively safe use of chemicals in industry, or as agrochemical, drugs, household chemicals or cosmetics. However, large numbers of laboratory animals have been used and distress has been caused to many of these animals [3].

This has led to extensive discussions on the ethical, scientific and financial feasibility of the current process of toxicity testing. As early as 1959, Russell and Burch[4] published their book "The Principles of Humane Experimental Technique" in which they introduced the terms Replacement, Reduction and Refinement, now commonly referred to as the 3 Rs. Since then, societal and political discussion has led to a number of legal regulations concerning the "humane" use of animals in experimentation in many countries as well as at the international level, e.g. within the European Community [5]. This does not mean, however, that these discussions have resulted in absolute consensus. On the one hand the animal protection movements maintain their objective that an end should be made to all animal experimentation, while on the other hand a major part of our society accepts such experiments as a necessity for e.g. scientific development or improved medical treatment. If human pharmacology and toxicology are considered, man is the most appropriate species of study. However, it is obvious for ethical reasons that a compound for which no data exist on its biological activity cannot be tested in man. Therefore, there is still a heavy reliance on laboratory animals as experimental models. However, ethical considerations apply also to the use of animals: animal studies should be justified and the alternatives that are available should be carefully considered [6].

Besides the ethical objections against the use of animals, there is also a scientific motivation for criticising the heavy reliance on animal data in toxicology. The use of animal data to predict the biological activities of compounds in humans is always prone to some degree of uncertainty. Important sources of uncertainty can be found in qualitative or quantitative differences between, for example, physiological and biochemical processes in animals and humans. As an example, the existence of differences in body size between the rat and humans implies a different ratio between body weight and body volume, resulting in different metabolic needs. The extrapolation of dose levels, calculated per kg body weight can therefore result in erroneous predictions with regard to the metabolism of the compound under study. Compound-specific parameters regarding uptake, distribution, biotransformation and excretion may also differ in a qualitative way [7]. These deviations may result in dissimilarities in the concentration of a compound at the target tissue. There can also be wide species differences in the modes of toxic action of compounds. Other difficulties arise from the fact that extrapolations have to be made from a rather small, but homogeneous, group of laboratory animals to the very heterogeneous human general population. In risk assessment for chemicals, toxicologists have traditionally attempted to overcome these uncertainties by introducing safety factors. For example, no-observed- (toxic) effect levels (NOELS) determined from animal experiments are divided by safety factors to account for interspecies and/or inter-individual differences in establishing safety standards for human exposure [1].

Non-animal test methods

Over the last decades an increasing number of test systems for evaluating the possible toxicological hazard of chemical compounds have been developed. Many of these systems do not rely on the use of intact animals, but make use of biological systems on a lower level of organisation than the organism: isolated organs, cell cultures, subcellular systems. These *in vitro* systems have been extremely useful in studying the molecular basis of a chemical's biological activity, including its mechanism(s) of toxic action. [8] Other important developments have been achieved in the prediction of biological reactivity on the basis of a compound's physico-chemical properties, such as structure, molecular size, reactive groups, etc.[9]. One application of this knowledge is in the construction of structure-activity relationships.

Knowledge on a compound's mechanism of toxic action either derived from *in vitro* systems or based on its structure can be the basis of hazard identification. Especially in the pharmaceutical and cosmetics industry a wide range of such approaches are being applied, mainly for screening purposes. However, the assessment of its risks cannot easily be made without further knowledge the compound's behaviour in the integrated system of an intact organism.

The ECITTS Scheme

In 1991, the European Research Group for Alternatives in Toxicity Testing (ERGATT), with the support of the Swedish Board for Laboratory Animals (CFN), established a multi-centre research project aimed at a more structured employment of non-animal methods to assess the toxicological properties of chemicals [10,11]. Important premises of this scheme were the desire to reduce the use of animals in standard toxicity testing, and to utilise the progress made in *in vitro* toxicology methods to test the toxic potency for selected cell types and tissues [12,13]. It is now generally recognised that the use of *in vitro* test systems is of particular interest in the study of mechanisms of toxic action. Knowledge of these mechanisms will also be a prerequisite for a more rational approach to toxic-logical hazard assessment [14,15]. Most attention is usually focused on the use of intact cells systems.

The ERGATT/CFN Integrated Toxicity Test Scheme (ECITTS) is based on the idea that sets of test batteries for predicting various types of local and systemic toxicity can be combined into integrated testing schemes that might be used to approach more comprehensive toxicity profiles for compounds. It is assumed that an "elementary analysis" of a compound's toxicity may be a more efficient approach to toxicity testing and hazard assessment, than animal-based investigations. "Elementary analysis" of toxicity would imply that the mode of toxic action of a compound can be broken down into a number of biokinetic and cellular events, each of which can be identified and quantified in appropriate model systems.

Results obtained from *in vitro* studies in general are often not directly applicable to the *in vivo* situation. One of the most obvious differences between the situation *in vitro* and *in vivo* is the absence of processes regarding absorption, distribution, metabolism and excretion (i.e. biokinetics) that govern the exposure of the target tissue of the organism *in vivo* [14,16]. The concentrations to which *in vitro* systems are exposed may not correspond to the actual situation at the target tissue after *in vivo* exposure. In addition, the occurrence of metabolic activation and/or saturation of specific metabolic pathways may also become relevant for the toxicity of a compound *in vivo* and this may lead to misinterpretation of *in vitro* data if such information is not taken into account. Therefore, predictive studies on biological activity of compounds require the integration of data on the mechanisms of action with data on biokinetic behaviour. Over the last decade, the feasibility of using mathematical models for interpretation of *in vivo* biokinetics has grown substantially [17]. This development has been facilitated by the increasing availability of computer-based techniques for numerical solution of differential equation sets that characterise biokinetic processes [18].

The aim of the ECITTS programme is the further development of the approach towards the prediction of possible toxicity of chemicals by integrating the knowledge obtained with non-animal studies (e.g. *in vitro* toxicity) with the application of physiologically-based biokinetic models, also to be parameterised from *in vitro* and other non-animal techniques. These toxicological profiles will be compared with known *in vivo* toxicity data in order to evaluate the validity of the approach.

The ECITTS scheme is very extensive and cannot be completed as a single project. Different aspects must therefore be investigated sequentially. Nevertheless, any study carried out in this scheme should comprise an examination of the fundamental ideas of ECITTS. In a first pilot study, the basal cytotoxicity, the *in vitro* neurotoxicity, in combination with a biokinetic analysis of five chemicals was studied [19]. From this study it became clear that a full biokinetic analysis might be difficult to achieve because of the limited availability of data in the field of *in vitro* biotransformation for many compounds.

The nervous system is highly susceptible to toxic insults. Observations indicating a role for environs-mental contaminants in neurodegenerative diseases and ageing, and incidents related to drug abuse, are contributing to the increasing societal awareness of the vulnerability of the nervous system to toxic insult. Due to the complexity and relative inaccessibility of the nervous system, cell culture studies have been of major importance in neuroscience research. However, there are no recommendations yet for the incorporation of alternative models into regulatory testing of neurotoxicity, as stated in the report on *in vitro* neurotoxicity testing [20]. The complexity and diversity of the nervous system also emphasize the importance of assessing neurotoxic insult *in vitro* by using a variety of test systems, with endpoints that consider the effect of chemicals both on general metabolic and specific neurochemical processes. The aim of this study was to represent an approach to prevalidate certain *in vitro* systems in the assessment of neurotoxicity.

In the currently described part of the ECITTS scheme, further investigations have been carried out as an extension of the first pilot study. Eight chemicals, with a documented effect on the nervous system ranging from low to high activity, were selected from the ECITTS list of reference chemicals [10]. *In vitro* studies of both general and specific aspects of neurotoxicity were performed on these chemicals, in parallel with determinations of their metabolism in *in vitro* liver models. The data on biotransformation were subsequently used in modelling the bio-kinetic behaviour of the compounds. From these data, the "target tissue" concentration (i.e. the brain concentration) in relation to different dosages of a compound could be modelled. A comparison with data on the biokinetics of the compound, as known from *in vivo* studies from the literature, enabled a validation of this approach.

Subsequently, the neurotoxic concentrations estimated in the applied *in vitro* systems were compared with the brain concentrations simulated by the model, thus also enabling a comparison of the toxic dose known from the literature, and the "dose" causing neuro-toxicity estimated from the models. The approach is more elaborately explained in the next paragraph.

9.2 Integration of kinetic and dynamic data to estimate systemic toxicity.

In order to allow a comparison between *in vitro* critical concentrations for the effects of a certain compound and the toxic dose for an intact organism, it is necessary to take into account the kinetic behaviour of the compound. The following scheme illustrates how this can be done.

1. The construction of a biokinetic model (for a certain compound; in a particular organism) depends on the availability of values for a number of parameters. Two different sets of parameters are needed: (a) physiological characteristics of the organism under study, and (b) physico-chemical characteristics of the compound. Building such a model on the basis of non-animal data will require data on the uptake, distribution, metabolism and excretion of the compound. A number of these parameters for metabolism can be determined in cell culture systems (e.g. biotransformation data obtained in hepatocyte cultures) or in sub-cellular systems (e.g. microsomes) [21]. Other cellular systems can be used to determine uptake rates and elimination rates (e.g. by measuring the transport rates over a cellular layer in cultures). Other useful data are the physico-chemical properties of the compounds, especially for predicting the distribution of compounds in the organism [22]. In many cases the applica-

tion of QSARs based on these properties allows a good estimation of transport and distribution. Biokinetic models can be constructed for animals as well as for man.

2. Once a biokinetic model has been constructed, its validity can be evaluated by comparing the predicted outcome of the model with the kinetics of the compound *in vivo*.
3. Since it will not always be possible (yet) to construct a biokinetic model solely based on *in vitro* data, another possibility is to incorporate kinetic parameters obtained in an *in vivo* experiment. In the framework of the ECITTS scheme this may be considered in those cases where the kinetics of low - non-toxic - doses can be extrapolated to the situation where it is applicable in the estimation of toxic effects. Physiologically based biokinetic models allow for these extrapolations. Such an exercise would also help in the construction of better *in vitro* models to measure the appropriate parameters. The measurement of uptake from the gastro-intestinal system after oral dosage is an example.
4. The desired outcome of a biokinetic model would be an estimation of the tissue concentration of the compound under study, especially in those targets that can be considered as the "target tissues" for the compound's biological activity. As an example, in the study described here the target tissue can be expected to be the central or the peripheral nervous system.
5. In parallel with kinetic studies, the toxic effects of a compound can be studied in *in vitro* or in other non-animal systems. For a good integration of all data it is essential that the appropriate test systems are available. This requires a thorough knowledge of the physiology of the target organs, and of the possible mechanisms of toxic action. When these prerequisites are fulfilled (i.e. when the appropriate parameters can be quantified in a non-animal system), then an estimate of the dynamics (e.g. as a critical active concentration) *in vitro* can be made. In our study, the measurement of parameters in a battery of cell cultures derived from the nervous system was selected, taking into account a number of possible neurotoxic (or neuro-active) mechanisms [20]. For a good interpretation of the results from these *in vitro* systems, the construction of concentration-effect relation-ships is necessary, since this allows the most accurate estimation of *in vivo* response surrogates or related "bench-marks", such as a concentration giving 20% of the maximal effect (EC20).
6. Integration of the kinetic and dynamic data will allow the prediction of the dynamics of a compound in an intact organism by means of using these response surrogates. Ideally, this would lead to the estimation of a "dose" that in an *in vivo* situation would result in those target tissue concentrations that are capable of giving a particular toxic effect.

7. From these data an estimate of ("surrogate") doses and related responses for minimal toxicity can be made. This can be expressed in the form of an "LOEL", "NOEL" or an EC20, but here too the most information can be extracted from "dose"-response curves. This can be done for different dosing regimes, e.g. relevant for acute or chronic toxicity, oral, inhalation or dermal dosage, etc.
8. Finally, the validity of the procedure for estimating the systemic toxicity of the compound under study can be evaluated by comparing the results with data obtained in an *in vivo* experiment.

Figure 1 gives a schematic representation of the different steps as described in more detail in these eight points.

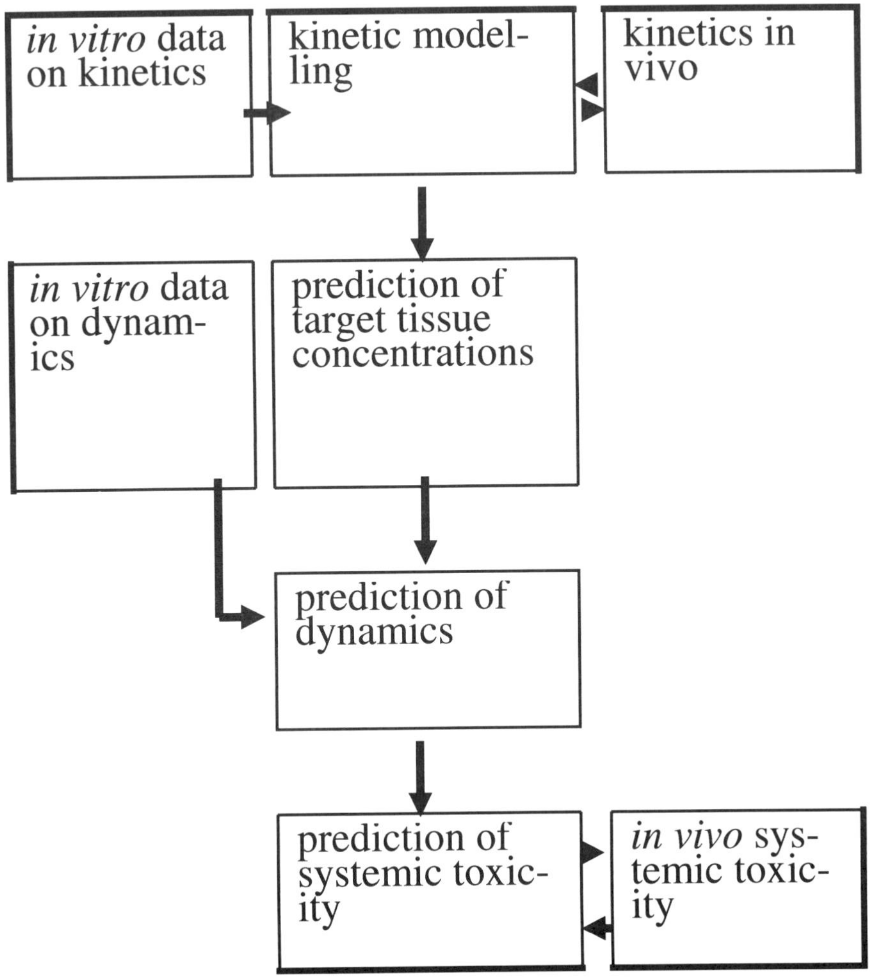

Figure 1. Schematic representation of the building blocks of activities for the integration of bio-kinetic and *in vitro*-derived biological effect parameters.

9.3 Biokinetic modelling

Biokinetic modelling describes the absorption, distribution, metabolism and elimination of xenobiotics as a function of dose and time within an organism. Biokinetic models can be divided into two main classes: databased compartmental models and physiologically-based compartmental models [23].

Databased compartmental models are the "classical" type of models in which the body usually is represented by a system that describes uptake, distribution, including inter-compartmental exchange, metabolism and excretion. The corresponding model parameters can be estimated by fitting the model to the data. The model parameter that describes the extent of distribution of the compound between blood or plasma and the other tissues is the apparent volume of distribution (Vd). This parameter, as well as the parameters on inter-compartmental diffusion rates, does not represent the actual tissue volumes, blood flows and diffusion rates in the body [24], but are the result of all processes regarding distribution, perfusion and diffusion. Due to the simplicity of databased models and the limited number of parameters, a model structure can be rapidly established and parameterised on the basis of the results of *in vivo* studies. However, com-part-mental models are merely descriptive of the data, they do not allow rationalisation of the mechanisms governing the kinetic processes.

The second class of biokinetic models, the physiologically based biokinetic (PB-BK) models, describe the compartments with respect to the known anatomy and physiology of the organism. Compartments correspond to relevant anatomical structures such as liver or kidney or tissue types such as fat or muscle. Tissue volumes and blood flow rates can either be determined experimentally or may be available from the literature [25]. The distribution of a compound throughout the body is described by tissue-blood partition coefficients. Metabolism and elimination of a compound can be described by either a linear clearance rate and/or a saturable Michaelis-Menten term in the liver or other organs capable of bio-transformation (e.g. the lung). The pulmonary ventilation rate and blood-air partition coefficient play a role in the uptake and exhalation of volatile compounds. These species-specific and compound-specific parameters form part of a set of differential equations that describe the biokinetic behaviour of a compound by means of a PB-BK model. The main advantage of PB-BK models over "classical" data-based compartmental models is their ability to estimate kinetic behaviour on the basis of a predetermined model structure produced using independently derived parameters, thereby omitting the need for any adjustment of the model parameters to create a "data fit". When biologically based descriptors are assigned to each of the specific kinetic processes, it becomes transparent that the distribution, metabolism and excretion of a compound are independent of the exposure route once the compound is taken up in the systemic circulation. Thus, it is possible to extrapolate from one exposure route to another by re-parameterising only the relevant uptake process, as the description of the distribution and elimination processes remains valid. Besides route-to-route extrapolation, the biologically based approach of PB-BK models also allows for extrapolation of dose and animal species beyond the conditions of laboratory studies [23].

Over the last ten years, the feasibility of this modelling approach has been greatly increased due to the availability of computer techniques that allow for the simultaneous, numerical solution of differential equations [26]. While many species-specific anatomical and physiological data have become available from the literature [27], compound-specific parameters for PB-BK models, like tissue-blood partition coefficients and the Michaelis-Menten constants Vmax and Km, are often still obtained by fitting these parameters to experimental data obtained *in vivo*. Proper use of PB-BK models in itself can contribute to replacement, reduction and refinement of animal studies by optimisation of study design through identification of critical parameters and timeframes in kinetic behaviour. In addition to this, incorporation *in vitro*-derived parameters will lead to a further reduction of large-scale animal studies for quantitative assessment of the biological activity of xenobiotics.

9.4 *In vitro* and other non-animal studies for obtaining compound-specific parameters for the use in PB-BK models

One of the main goals of the ECITTS project was to study the feasibility of obtaining PB-BK model parameters exclusively from *in vitro* or other non-animal techniques in order to estimate the biokinetics of compounds *in vivo*. A number of elements need special attention and will be considered in more detail: absorption, distribution on the basis of partitioning of the compound, and metabolism.

Absorption

Absorption forms the first step in the sequence of interactions between a compound and the organism. If a compound is administered parenterally, the description of direct infusion into the venous blood stream is straightforward. However, the absorption of compounds by occupational or environmental exposure is seldom parenteral but usually oral, dermal or via inhalation. Although the biological complexity of *in vivo* absorption processes complicates the application of *in vitro* models, some techniques have been developed to estimate oral and dermal absorption processes from *in vitro* test systems [28,29,30,31]. In addition, attempts have been undertaken to describe oral and dermal absorption by quantitative structure activity relationships [32,33,34]. In general, application of these predictive systems has been limited to series of structurally related homologues.

Tissue-blood partitioning

Tissue-air partition coefficients (PCs) of volatile compounds can be measured *in vitro* by incubation of the compound with a homogenate of the respective tissue in buffered saline. The equilibrium distribution of the compound is then measured by gas-chromatographic analysis of the air present in the headspace of the vial containing the homogenate/buffer mixture [35,36,37]. Tissue-blood partition coefficients can be calculated by dividing the tissue-air PCs by the respective blood-air PCs. This method has been applied in many studies on volatile hydrocarbons with human and rat blood, liver, lung, kidney, fat, muscle, and brain homogenates [37,38]. This principle has been extended to tissue-blood PCs of non-volatile compounds by the use of a number of *in vitro* methods that are based on the incubation of compounds with a buffered tissue homogenate [39,40]. In addition to these *in vitro* techniques, both descriptive and mechanistic algorithms for estimation of blood-air and tissue-blood partition coefficients have been reported [22]. All methods attempt to estimate the biological partitioning process as a function of non-biological data such as water and/or lipid solubility of a compound.

The distribution rate of a compound to the brain may be described mathematically as a function of input into the brain from the arterial blood stream and outflow from the venous side. Assumption of a venous equilibration model implies that the concentration of a compound in the venous blood leaving the brain is always in equilibrium with that in the brain tissue. This model can expected to be valid for small nonpolar, lipophilic as well as hydro-philic compounds. Thus, the perfusion rate of the brain dominates over the diffusion rate through the blood-brain barrier as the rate-limiting step in brain distribution. Depending on chemical structure, other compounds may express a diffusion limited brain uptake *in vivo*, requiring a compound-specific parameter for diffusion rate. In the case of polar and/or ionised compounds, an energy-dependent, saturable uptake rate, similar to the Michaelis-Menten description of metabolism, may be required to describe its interaction with the blood brain barrier.

Metabolism

Several *in vitro* techniques have been applied based on incubation of the test compound with tissue homogenates, cell suspensions or subcellular fractions such as microsomes [21,41,42]. In this respect, the liver is the most studied organ but extra-hepatic metabolism kinetics, e.g. of lung tissue, have also been reported [43]. Special test systems have been developed for volatile organics *in vitro* [44,45]. Depending on the occurrence of metabolic activation and subsequent covalent binding, either the disappearance of parent compound or the formation rate of specific metabolites may be relevant for analysis of the role of kinetics in the toxicity of a compound.

The recent notable success [21] in relating the rate of *in vitro* metabolism of several compounds with the corresponding events *in vivo* represents a major step as traditionally the value of *in vitro* metabolising systems was considered to be purely qualitative in nature. The basis of this relationship is the use of the parameter, intrinsic clearance, which is a pure measure of enzyme activity towards a compound *in vivo* and is not influenced by other physiological determinants of clearance such as hepatic blood flow or drug binding. This parameter has an *in vitro* equivalent as it corresponds to the Vmax:Km ratio. The utility of *in vitro* intrinsic clearance as a predictor of *in vivo* intrinsic clearance, and hence hepatic clearance and total body clearance has been assessed with a database of 35 drug substrates for rat cytochrome P450 [46].

The value of *in vitro* : *in vivo* extrapolation is clearly demonstrated by considering kinetic data from incubations with freshly isolated hepatocytes. The determination of easily measurable *in vitro* parameters, such as Vmax and Km from initial rate studies, and scaling from the *in vitro* situation by accounting for the hepatocellularity, provides *in vivo* intrinsic clearance estimates. A scaling factor of 110 million cells per gram of liver has proven to be a robust parameter independent of laboratory technique and insensitive to animal pre-treatment with various inducers and inhibitors, which alter cytochrome P450 complement and zonal distribution of isozymes. Similar procedures can also be adopted for other *in vitro* systems such as hepatic microsomes and liver slices. An appropriate scaling factor for microsomal studies is the microsomal recovery index, which allows for the incomplete recovery of cytochrome P450 with standard differential centrifugation of liver homogenates. This scaling factor averages 45mg microsomal protein per gram of liver, but is laboratory dependent, influenced by animal pre-treatments and hence, unlike hepatocellularity, must be individualized for laboratory/study. Using the database, micro-somal prediction has proved "successful" in two-thirds of cases, whilst for hepatocyte data "successful" predictions have been achieved in 90% of cases. Success is defined by a predicted/observed intrinsic clearance ratio of between 0.5-2. The hepatocellularity of a liver slice has not been a satisfactory parameter for scaling kinetic data from liver slices. The level of success varies from compound to compound and diffusion of substrate is a competing process to metabolism within the slice incubation system. Hence low clearance compounds are better predicted than high clearance compounds. The use of three liver models (venous equilibration, parallel tube and dispersion) has been compared to predict hepatic clearance from *in vitro* intrinsic clearance values. No consistent advantage of one model over others could be demonstrated. Thus, the simplest venous equilibration model appears adequate for the currently available data in hepatocytes and microsomes [21].

While these successes are extremely encouraging as they establish the fidelity of *in vitro* systems for *in vivo* prediction, the level of success varies from compound to compound. It is important to address the reasons for failure of prediction by each *in vitro* system and it is noteworthy that the current approach simplifies several key issues. Three key issues have been identified which would limit the applicability of the *in vitro* metabolic approach to both PB-BK modelling and metabolic stability screening in general. These are:

- Extension of the intrinsic clearance approach to compounds which display sigmoidal enzyme kinetics. This type of kinetics is now known to be a characteristic of the most abundant CYP in human liver, CYP3A4.
- The use of a time course for substrate depletion as an alternative to Vmax:Km determination of compounds where metabolic fate has not been extensively characterized. Questions arising in the use of this approach include - which sample should be analysed (whole incubate, separate cells or media), the effect of media binding and the impact of prolonged metabolite production.
- The role of product inhibition in hepatic microsomes due to non-functional phase-II metabolism.

Implementation in the ECITTS programme

In the ECITTS study research was carried out to resolve these generic issues in order to aid the modelling procedures in general and to increase the credibility of the scaling procedure. Eight model compounds were selected for evaluating the approach described above: benzene, toluene, lindane, acrylamide, parathion/oxon, diazepam, caffeine and phenytoin. The nervous system is considered to be the target tissue for these compounds. In addition to *in vitro-in vivo* extrapolations, some attempts have been made to correlate the metabolic rate constants of a series of halogenated methanes and ethanes with their chemical structure [47]. Reasonable correlations were obtained for compounds that are exclusively metabolised by a particular isoform of the cytochrome P450 super family. However, the predictive power of such techniques should be interpreted with caution, since the mechanistic significance of molecular descriptors for the metabolic process may be very dependent on the specific chemical structure of the homologues that are studied, and the enzyme/isoform(s) involved in their metabolism. Considerably more studies are required on *in vitro-in vivo* extrapolation before predictions from chemical structure are a serious reality.

9.5 Toxicity test batteries: *in vitro* approaches

Next to the biokinetic considerations, the evaluation of a compound's toxicity is another important step in the procedure described in figure 1. In the ECITTS programme we focused on eight compounds with a known neurotoxic character. Therefore, we here will consider the approach for measuring the neurotoxicity of the compounds in a battery of *in vitro* neurotoxicity tests.

Strategies for how a test battery for neurotoxicity determination *in vitro* should be constituted have been proposed elsewhere [48,49,50]. It was suggested that testing should be performed in stepwise procedures as shown in the simplified scheme below.

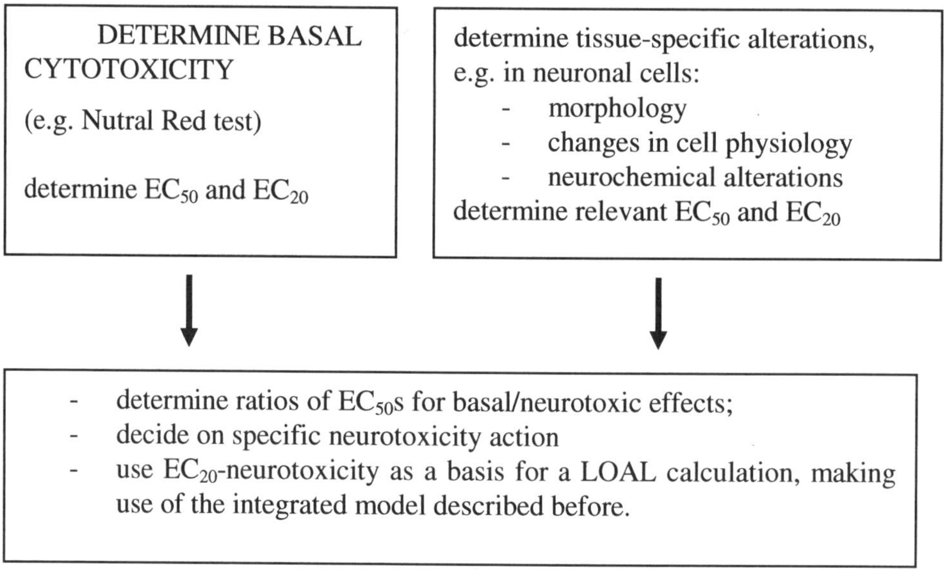

Figure 2. Scheme for the determination of relevant neurotoxic effects of compounds.

Biokinetics, physico-chemical data and *in vivo* information (where available) of the test compounds, should also be included in the test strategy.

The proposed test schemes were based on established cell lines as well as on highly differentiated primary cultures of neuronal cells and glial cells. In the ECITTS study human neuroblastoma SH-SY5Y cells were used, which were differentiated by retinoic acid (RA). The advantage of human cells, as opposed to other mammalian cells, is that they correlate better to human toxicity [51]. Nevertheless, the mouse fibroblast 3T3 cell line was used for determination of basal cytotoxicity.

The endpoints investigated in this study were selected according to the stepwise procedure for the identification of neurotoxicants. All effects were detected after 72 hours of exposure with the ECITTS reference chemicals. The basal cytotoxicity was determined by measuring the total cellular protein content. Morphological alterations were observed and neurite degeneration quantified. The neurite per cell ratio was used as a marker for axonopathy [52]. Cell physiology was measured in terms of protein synthesis rate and calcium homeostasis (i.e. the basal intracellular free calcium concentration, [Ca2+]i) [53]. The protein synthesis rate was measured as a general marker of cellular metabolism, but may also reflect effects on gene expression (general inhibition of transcription or translation) [54]. The calcium homeostasis was studied because of the prerequisite of maintaining a low basal [Ca2+]i for functional signal transduction and signal transmission [55], as well as for Ca2+-dependent processes as mediators of neurotoxicity [56], and the role of Ca2+ in cell death [57,58]. The neurochemical functions studied were KCl-induced Ca2+-influx through voltage-operated calcium channels (VOCC) because of the importance of precise pre-synaptic ion-gated Ca2+ currents for neuronal transmission, and effects on muscarinic acetylcholine receptor (mAChR)-activated Ca2+-fluxes because of the role of G-protein coupled receptors in neuronal signal transduction and modulation. Retinoic acid-differentiated SH-SY5Y cells express mAChRs, linked to the inositol 1,4,5-trisphosphate (IP3) second messenger pathway [59], they develop VOCC [60] as well as an extensive network of neurites [61]. Therefore, the cells serve as a suitable model for studies of the neuronal functions selected in this investigation and no primary cultures of different species (e.g. rat) needed to be included in the test battery.

The critical cellular neurotoxic concentration (CNC) is determined for each compound. CNC is equal to the concentration that causes 20% effect, as compared to unexposed control cells (EC20), in the most sensitive endpoint in the test battery. Where no concentration-effect curve can be determined, CNC is equal to the lowest concentration that induces a statistically significant effect as compared to control cells (LOEC).

9.6 Results of the ECITTS project

As is indicated in the scheme in fig 1, the results of this study will need to be evaluated in two different ways:

1. the outcome of the biokinetic modelling, based on the *in vitro* and other non-animal studies can be compared with data of the kinetics of the compounds *in vivo*;

2. the systemic toxicity data as predicted on the basis of the biokinetic modelling and on *in vitro* toxicity testing can be compared with *in vivo*-derived data on systemic toxicity.

The outcome of this evaluation can conveniently be grouped for compounds with a similar behaviour. We here consider four situations:
- volatile organic compounds,
- persistent lipophilic pesticides; lindane and parathion/paraoxon.
- pharmaceuticals & food components,
- reactive chemicals

1) KINETIC *IN VITRO-IN VIVO* EXTRAPOLATIONS

Volatile organic compounds (VOCs); benzene & toluene.
The results for these compounds [62] demonstrate the feasibility of the *in vitro*-derived metabolic parameters of benzene for simulation of *in vivo* metabolism. It may be concluded that application of the three sets of *in vitro* data, derived from either microsomal or S-9 homogenate incubation by the vial equilibration method, resulted in acceptable simulations of benzene's metabolism *in vivo*. For simulation of benzene's brain-blood PC in the rat, QSARs may be used. In addition, a human brain-blood PC has been reported. Due to the absence of studies on brain uptake of benzene *in vivo*, validity of this aspect could not be evaluated.

In vitro-to-*in vivo* extrapolation of toluene's metabolism was successfully performed [63]. The results from data using intact *in situ* perfused livers did not lead to a more accurate simulation of toluene's disposition *in vivo* than did application of freshly isolated S-9 homogenate. Biotransformation data, derived from incubation in a reconstituted microsomal system, resulted in a rather unrealistic Km value. The fact that product formation was monitored, as opposed to substrate disappearance of substrate in all other studies, makes it difficult to compare application of such a system with other *in vitro* systems used for assessing toluene's metabolism. The brain-blood partition coefficient of toluene was slightly over-estimated. Direct determination of this parameter using a rat brain homogenate resulted in a value of 1.1, as opposed to the value of 2.0 that was estimated beforehand by us, and values of 1.2-1.6 that were eventually derived from the *in vivo* studies used in the evaluation.

For both benzene and toluene, simulations of brain concentrations following acute inhalation exposure were feasible on the basis of a fully *in vitro*-based PB-PK model. Since both compounds show rapid metabolism and perfusion-limited distribution, simulation of (sub)chronic, intermittent exposure (e.g. 8 hr/day for a 7 day period), does not result in accumulation in the brain over a multi-day exposure period. This presently limits the estimation the toxicity of benzene and toluene in acute exposure scenarios.

persistent lipophilic pesticide: lindane and parathion/paraoxon.
No *in vitro* data on lindane's biotransformation were available from the literature [64]. Tissue-blood PCs were available for liver, fat and muscle (i.e. slowly perfused) tissue. The blood-fat PC reported *in vitro* was approximately one hundred and this is about two-fold lower than observed after chronic exposure *in vivo*. Obviously, fat is not a target tissue in itself. However, for lipophilic compounds like lindane, a major part of the total body burden is present in the fat compartment. Thus, blood and brain concentrations become inversely related to the fat-blood PC. The brain-blood PC was initially derived from an *in vivo* study. Estimation of lindane's brain-blood PC from its Kow, using a QSAR, lead to a value that was very similar to the value observed in the *in vivo* studies. Besides the parameters for metabolism and partitioning, the oral uptake rate is also a relevant parameter for *in vivo* exposure to lindane. This parameter was derived from *in vivo* studies, as no appropriate *in vitro*, or other non-animal techniques were available.

The PB-PK model could eventually be calibrated by a mixture of *in vitro*-(fat, liver, muscle PCs), QSAR- (brain PC) and *in vivo*-derived (metabolism and oral uptake) parameters. Using this model, simulation of lindane brain levels, following both acute and (sub)chronic exposures, could be evaluated and proved to be feasible.

For biotransformation of parathion into its active metabolite paraoxon, four sets of *in vitro*-derived biotransformation parameters were available [e.g. 65]. A single, *in vitro*-derived, rate constant was available for paraoxon hydrolysis. *In vitro*-derived PCs were available for fat, liver and muscle tissue for both compounds. The brain-blood PC for paraoxon had to be derived from its Kow, on the basis of a QSAR. Oral, i.p. and s.c. uptake rates for parathion were neither available from *in vivo* studies nor from *in vitro*, or other non-animal, techniques. Thus, the PB-PK model was eventually parameterised by a mixture of *in vitro* (metabolism and fat, liver, muscle PCs) and QSAR (paraoxon brain-blood PC) techniques. Simulations of parathion tissue levels, following acute i.v. exposure to parathion showed that parathion concentrations in fat could not be adequately estimated due to the apparent occurrence of diffusion-limited uptake and release *in vivo*. In addition, parathion liver concentrations were systematically underpredicted using three of the four available datasets of *in vitro*-derived metabolic parameters. However, parathion brain concentrations were adequately estimated.

Results for paraoxon, the active metabolite, are more relevant for parathion toxicity. Simulation of paraoxon plasma levels, based on the *in vitro*-derived hydrolysis rate were compared to experimental results obtained after direct i.v. injection of the metabolite itself, was successful. Simulations of paraoxon brain levels resulting from i.v. dosage of parathion were comparable to the experimental results. However, this does not necessarily imply that the simulations of paraoxon brain concentration after dosing with parathion can unequivocally be considered reliable. Firstly, the value of the experimental data on paraoxon brain levels is limited as concentrations were followed for up to one hour only. In addition, the errors observed in the simulations of liver concentrations of parathion, and also paraoxon, indicate general shortcomings in either the model structure and/or in the *in vitro*-derived parameters for metabolism of parathion to paraoxon. The occurrence of diffusion limited fat-blood distribution may even enhance this effect. If the diffusion limitations of fat-blood distribution are accounted for properly, this could result in higher amounts of parathion available for hepatic metabolism. A conclusive answer to the present uncertainties regarding parathion and paraoxon kinetics requires a sensitivity analysis on a set of model parameters that are optimised to an experimental dataset that is more comprehensive than the presently available one.

pharmaceuticals & food components: caffeine, phenytoin and diazepam.
In vivo and *in vitro* biotransformation of caffeine, phenytoin and diazepam are discussed in appendix 6 of [66]. The *in situ* perfused liver, as reported in one study, appears to give the best estimation of caffeine metabolism *in vivo.* In contrast, another study that used this method, reported Vmax values that are approximately four-fold lower than the values derived *in vivo.* Studies from either microsomal or hepatocyte incubation of caffeine reported Vmax and Km values that were both overestimated in comparison with the *in vivo* data. The Vmax/Km ratio derived *in vitro*, representing linear clearance under unsaturated conditions, can be considered acceptable, provided that realistic substrate concentrations have been used *in vitro.* Estimation of the brain-blood PC by our QSAR resulted in an acceptable value as compared with the value derived from the *in vivo* studies.

For phenytoin, an occurrence of product inhibition of metabolism is observed both *in vitro* and *in vivo.* In the *in vitro*-to-*in vivo* extrapolation, this phenomenon may be taken into account by application of a descriptive relationship, e.g. between Vmax or Cli and the initial plasma or medium concentration of the substrate (appendix 10 of [66]). A more preferable approach would be to establish a sub model on hepatic levels of the metabolite following identification of either a competitive, non-competitive or uncompetitive inhibition concept *in vitro.* This approach is presently under study, but the reported mechanistic descriptions of inhibition [66-7] could not be used in the results due to difficulties in obtaining *in vitro* data on clearance of phenytoin's main metabolite. Brain-blood distribution of phenytoin was estimated by QSAR, resulting in a 2-3-fold underestimation of its PC reported *in vivo*.

The metabolic clearance rate of diazepam *in vivo* has been reported to vary approximately 4-fold among the different studies. Although product inhibition of diazepam metabolism, similar to that for phenytoin, has been shown, a dependency of clearance rates on applied dose or initial medium concentrations was not observed. When comparing diazepam clearance rates that were reported *in vitro* and *in vivo* within a single study, using the same experimental conditions, it may be concluded that microsomal incubation can lead to adequate estimation of *in vivo* clearance at low (< 1 mg/L) substrate concentrations. At higher concentrations, use of hepatocytes is considered to be preferable over microsomes. This confirms the role of product inhibition in the metabolism of diazepam. As may be expected, the use of hepatocytes in a cultured system, as opposed to a suspension, leads to a substantial underestimation of metabolic rate. This can be attributed to the general loss of cytochrome P450 activity that is reported to occur for cultured hepatocytes. Brain-blood distribution of diazepam was estimated by QSAR and resulted in a less than two-fold underestimation of its PC reported *in vitro*. Eventually, PB-PK models for all three compounds could be parameterised almost fully by application of the results of *in vitro* studies. Only oral and i.p. uptake parameters were derived from *in vivo* studies. Using these models, simulations of brain levels of all three compounds, following acute exposure, could be evaluated and generally proved to be feasible. Since all compounds show rapid metabolism and perfusion-limited distribution, simulation of (sub) chronic, daily exposure does not result in accumulation in the brain over the exposure period. This limits the estimation of toxicity to acute exposure scenarios.

reactive compounds: acrylamide.

In contrast with most other compounds considered in the present study, a classic 'compartmental' model was chosen for simulation of acrylamidc kinctics [68]. Thc small molccular size and high water-solubility of this compound motivated this choice. In addition, acrylamide's neurotoxicity is assumed to be expressed mainly through its action on the peripheral nervous system. Therefore, the brain-blood distribution of this compound was not considered and blood concentrations were assumed to be an appropriate measure for PNS exposure.

No *in vitro* data on biotransformation of acrylamide were available from the literature, and this information was derived from an *in vivo* study. In the 'classical' model structure selected for acrylamide, the distribution volume represents the resultant of distribution in the individual tissues, weighted by the respective partition coefficients. Based on acrylamide's water solubility, Vd was assumed to approximate total body water.

Thus, the model was eventually parameterised by a mixture of physiological (Vd) and *in vivo*-derived (metabolism and uptake rate) parameters. Simulation of blood levels, following both acute and (sub)chronic exposure could be evaluated and lead to acceptable simulations of acrylamide blood levels after acute and subchronic exposure reported in other studies.

2) TOXICITY: *IN VITRO-IN VIVO* EXTRAPOLATIONS

Volatile organic compounds (VOCs); benzene & toluene.
After extensive attempts, the neurotoxicity test battery eventually proved to be unsuitable for assessing the *in vitro* activity of benzene and toluene. This was mainly due to their volatility and their interaction with the plastic material required for cultivation of the cells.

Since adequate kinetic models for both compounds could be established [62,63]), an alternative approach was chosen to address the role of kinetics in the acute toxicity of these compounds [69]. In addition to benzene and toluene, a group of related (industrial) solvents, for which *in vitro*-derived kinetic model parameters are available, was also considered. Acute lethality and non-specific neurotoxicity were chosen as endpoints and a set of experimentally reported LC50 and EC30 exposure concentrations for these endpoints was retrieved from the literature. The kinetic model was used to simulate the concentrations in a theoretically motivated target tissue (brain lipid membranes) resulting from exposure to each compound at the respective LC50 or EC30 concentrations. It was observed that differences in solvent toxicity for acute and non-specific, narcosis related, endpoints, are explained by differences in kinetic behaviour. The onset of lethality for these compounds was found to correspond to a target tissue concentration of approximately 70 mM, regardless of the compound structure or length of exposure. The results of these studies allow for the estimation of acute lethal concentrations, or concentrations that affect sublethal neurotoxic endpoints. This approach is limited to non-reactive compounds that do not express their toxicity through mechanisms other than acute accumulation in the lipid membranes of CNS cells.

Thus, a priori estimation of benzene's and toluene's toxicity on the basis of *in vitro*-derived toxicity parameters was not feasible. However, *in vitro*-derived information on kinetic behaviour and literature data on *in vivo* toxicity has lead to the development of a tool for estimating acute toxicity of volatile organic compounds under the constraints discussed above.
persistent lipophilic pesticides; lindane and parathion/paraoxon

Combining the data on lindane's effect on voltage operated calcium channels in the *in vitro* neurotoxicity test battery with the kinetic model simulations, both acute and subchronic LOELs were estimated (appendix 21 in [66]. The results generally compared well to experimental LOELs reported for this compound in *in vivo* studies. Possible shortcomings are indicated by the difference between the estimated time for onset of effects and the time at which these effects actually occurred *in vivo*.

Combining the data on paraoxon's neuro-degenerative effect (appendix 16 in [66]) from the *in vitro* neurotoxicity test battery with the kinetic model simulations, a LOEL for acute paraoxon exposure was estimated (appendix 23 in [66]). Although the *in vitro* cytotoxicity for both parathion and paraoxon was also assessed by the Kenacid Blue Assay (appendix 17 in [66]), their activity in the latter test system was substantially smaller and was therefore not used for LOEL estimates. The estimated LOEL, based on neurite degeneration, was >2-fold higher than the experimentally reported LOEL. In addition, the estimated time of effect onset (48 hr) was substantially different from the observed time for the maximum effect (2 hr). Based on para-oxon's specific neuro-degenerative effect, a (sub)chronic LOEL could not be estimated. This has two main causes. Firstly, according to the kinetic model simulations, paraoxon does not accumulate *in vivo*. Secondly, the neurotoxicity test battery results for paraoxon did not include provision for a possible time-concentration-response relationship for paraoxon exposure, but only for a concentration-response relationship. For rapidly metabolized compounds that do not accumulate over time, *in vitro* concentration-response data limit the effect estimates to the time-window that corresponds with the actual presence of the compound in the target tissue, and thus to acute exposure situations. Situations where the half-life of the effect is larger than the half-life of the compound cannot be assessed without the availability of time-concentration-response data.

Alternatively, it was attempted to estimate paraoxon's subchronic LOEL on the basis of additional literature studies on AChE inhibition *in vitro*. The results underestimated an experimentally derived LOEL, based on the occurrence of clinical symptoms, by a factor of six.

pharmaceuticals & food components: caffeine, phenytoin and diazepam.
The most sensitive endpoint for caffeine's neurotoxicity was found to be its effect on voltage operated calcium channels (appendix 13 in [66]). A concentration-dependent response was not observed for this effect. This is thought to be the result of the occurrence of transient compensatory mechanisms occurring within the time frame of the exposure period, resulting in an apparently idiosyncratic concentration-response relation. (Multiple targets)

For phenytoin, the two most sensitive endpoints within the test battery were neurite degeneration and inhibition of protein synthesis rate (appendix 14 in [66]). In addition, effects on rat brain micromass cultures were also found to be sensitive to phenytoin exposure, as reported in the literature. Phenytoin's *in vitro* effects on sodium channels were also retrieved from the literature.

Diazepam's effect on voltage operated calcium channels was found to be one of the most sensitive effects within the test battery (appendix 15 in [66]). *In vitro* effects on sodium channels and y-aminobutyric acid (GABA) receptors were retrieved from the literature.

Due to the rapid biotransformation of all three compounds, accumulation in brain tissue does not occur following dosage once a day for a prolonged number of days. For the same reasons discussed before for paraoxon, it is therefore not possible to estimate LOELs for (sub)chronic exposure. Such estimates require information on the time-concentration-response relationships that are not available from the neurotoxicity test battery as it is presently implemented.

Behavioural parameters were found for all three compounds to be the most sensitive indicators for their activity *in vivo*. Most *in vivo* studies followed a dose-response design with at least three different doses. Therefore, EC20 values for *in vivo* activity could be derived after taking into account the relation between external dose and target tissue concentration with the kinetic model. For statistical reasons, such *in vivo*-derived EC20 values are preferred over LOEL values. Comparison between the *in vitro* EC20 (or) CNC values and the *in vivo*-derived values obviously shows that it is essential to use appropriate *in vitro* endpoints when making quantitative estimates about a compound's *in vivo* activity. Thus, the *in vivo* activity of phenytoin and diazepam could only be estimated adequately after consideration of *in vitro* assays on rat brain micromass cultures and GABA receptors, respectively. Both assays are presently not included in the neurotoxicity test battery.

reactive chemicals: acrylamide.

In the light of the previously discussed problems regarding (sub)chronic LOEL estimations for compounds for which the half-life of their effects are larger than their kinetic half-life (paraoxon, caffeine, phenytoin and diazepam), a new approach was attempted for acrylamide [68]. Its neurodegenerative effects were found to be the most sensitive endpoint within the *in vitro* test battery, and are considered most relevant for the neurodegenerative effects *in vivo*. Therefore, the *in vitro* effects of acrylamide were re-assessed under an exposure scenario with variable exposure lengths and a post-exposure recovery period. The resulting information was used to express effects as a function of both time and exposure concentration, including a measure for post-exposure recovery. After incorporation of the data into a simple kinetic model, LOELs for acute, 10, 30 and 90 day i.p. exposures were estimated, and agreed very well with experimental results.

In terms of quantitative and qualitative performance, the estimations for acrylamide are considered to be the most successful among the eight compounds considered in the present study.

In summary, the estimated and experimental LOELs for 6 of the 8 compounds considered in this part of the ECITTS study are compared (fig. 3). The discrepancy between estimated and experimental LOELs ranges from approximately a factor two, for compounds with a low toxicity (i.e. a high LOEL), to a factor 10, for compounds with a high toxicity (i.e. a low LOEL). Thus, LOEL estimates for compounds with a relatively low toxicity are more successful than the estimates for compounds with a relatively high toxicity. It should be noted (again) that LOELs of the most toxic compounds (diazepam, parathion and paraoxon) could only be established after consideration of *in vitro* test results that were derived form the literature. The specific toxicity of these compounds was not reflected by the endpoints within the *in vitro* neurotoxicity test battery. In addition, the results show that the LOEL estimations for acrylamide benefit from the extended testing protocol for this compound. For this compound we have extended the original neurotoxicity test battery protocol by establishing time-concentration-response relationships, including a post-exposure recovery period. In contrast with caffeine, phenytoin and diazepam, this extra information has allowed us to estimate the (sub)chronic toxicity with a high degree of accuracy.

9.7 Discussion

The results described above, both for the kinetic and for the dynamic aspects of the *in vitro-in vivo* extrapolation are encouraging with respect to the possibilities for the integration of these approaches in a toxicological risk assessment. However, there are a number remaining issues that will be discussed here.

9.7.1 Kinetics

The estimation of kinetic behaviour of compounds from data derived from non-animal methods is one of the two main goals of the ECITTS study. Basically, the issues that are to be discussed follow the basic processes that govern kinetic behaviour: absorption, distribution and elimination.

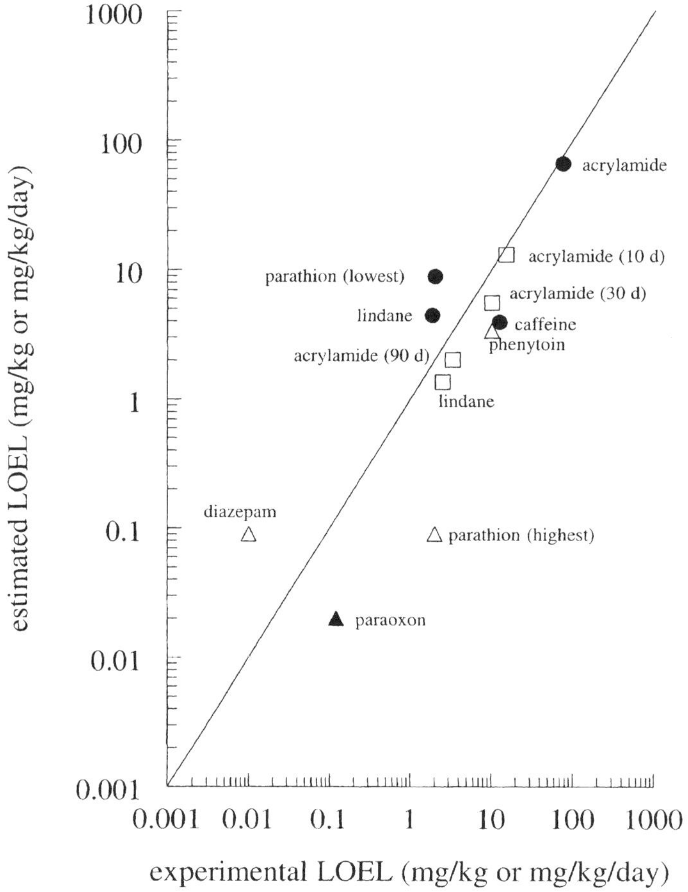

Figure 3. Comparison of experimental and estimated LOELs made in this study for six compounds.
• : acute LOELs estimated on the basis of the neurotoxicity test battery results
❑: (sub)chronic LOELs estimated on the basis of the neurotoxicity test battery results
▲: acute LOELs estimated on the basis of additional *in vitro* (literature) studies
Δ: (sub)chronic LOELs estimated on the basis of *in vitro* literature studies
The line represents identity (experimental = estimated)

Absorption
For the absorption of compounds, it can be concluded that pulmonary uptake of volatile compounds [62,63] can be adequately described by the physiologically motivated equilibration assumptions between alveolar air and blood that were originally reported for styrene [70]. Although both *in vitro* and QSAR-based techniques for quantification of oral and dermal uptake have

been reported, application of these methods has not been evaluated since no adequate data were available to us for the eight compounds within the present study. The QSAR algorithms that have been reported are commonly restricted to groups of chemical homologues that do not allow for a straightforward application to the chemicals of the present study [28,32,33,34,71]. In addition, comprehensive evaluation of such approaches requires the availability of data derived from *in vivo* studies. Thus, a preliminary inventory of available literature data on oral and dermal absorption aspects seems desirable when establishing the design of a possible follow-up of the present study. Although similar problems have been met during this study regarding the description of intraperitoneal and subcutaneous dosages these can be considered less significant, since these administration routes are usually limited to the laboratory situation, and are seldom required for the assessment of eventual human exposure and uptake.

Partition coefficients

Techniques for determination of tissue-blood and blood-air partition coefficients (PCs) of volatile compounds like benzene and toluene, are now well established [38] and the values retrieved from the literature could be readily incorporated into the kinetic models [62,63,64], (see also appendix 23 in [66]). When literature data are absent, the application of quantitative structure-activity, or property-property, relationships (QSAR/QPPRs) apparently offers a good alternative (appendix 6 in [66]). However, the level of detail by which these partition processes are presently described may be improved [22]. Other studies have brought up two key issues in this aspect: the dose-dependency of the blood binding, due to saturable binding sites on the haemoglobin, and the differential physico-chemical properties of neutral lipids and phospholipids in blood and tissues [72]. Further analysis of these aspects requires more tissue distribution data from the literature, as well as the generation of (quantum) chemical parameters in addition to the octanol/water and water/air PCs that are presently used as the descriptors for tissue distribution. For non-volatile compounds, the feasibility of QPPR/QSAR methods is even more significant. The presently available *in vitro* techniques for direct assessment of tissue-blood PCs require substantially more effort than for volatile compounds [39,40]. Here also, a comprehensive evaluation of the available literature should accompany the design of further studies in this field.

Model structure

In relation to the issues regarding the tissue-blood PCs the individual tissues, the results for paraoxon (appendix 23 in [66]) indicate that a 'classical', compartmental-based approach can some-times be used instead of a PB-PK model [73]. Full sensitivity analysis of a PB-PK model is required before possible simplifications of a model structure are to be considered. In general, it may be expected that small, uncharged and water-soluble compounds, with a hepatic clearance rate smaller than the liver perfusion rate, are the most likely candidates for such a model simplification. Caffeine is the most likely candidate for which a compartmental approach could work equally well as the presently exercised physiologically based-approach.

Scaling of biotransformation parameters
Regarding the application of *in vitro*-derived data for estimation of biotransformation *in vivo*, a number of issues explicitly arise from the present approach. There is a rather wide choice in available *in vitro* systems for quantitative assessment of hepatic biotransformation. The most commonly used systems are freshly isolated liver or S-9 homogenate, reconstituted microsomes and hepatocytes, either in culture or suspension. Although *in situ* perfused livers resemble the *in vivo* situation most closely, the sacrifice of a relatively large number of animals is required, and this method is obviously not applicable for assessment of human metabolism. For the present study, *in vitro*-derived biotransformation data were available for benzene, toluene, parathion, paraoxon, caffeine, phenytoin and diazepam. Comparison of *in vitro*- and *in vivo*-derived biotransformation data shows that kinetic simulations for benzene, toluene and caffeine generally led to adequate results on the basis of S-9 homogenate or microsome studies [62,63]. In contrast, studies reporting on hepatocyte suspensions were clearly superior to micro-somal studies for simulation of phenytoin and diazepam kinetics (appendix 6 in [66]). No *in vitro* data could be retrieved for lindane and acrylamide [64,68], and kinetic simulations for parathion and paraoxon could not be evaluated comprehensively in this aspect, due to the limited availability of more relevant data (appendix 23 in [66]). This poses questions on the judgement of the most appropriate *in vitro* system that is to be applied for kinetic model simulations in general. Obviously, application of microsomal systems is limited to compounds that undergo oxidative metabolism by the cytochrome P450 system. In addition, the results for phenytoin and diazepam indicate that the occurrence of product inhibition in the metabolism of compounds can also be a key factor in the inappropriate assessment of a compound's metabolism through microsomal systems (appendix 6, 7 & 10 in [66]. Prior prediction of the possible occurrence of product inhibition of a compound would require detailed knowledge of the nature of the inhibitory mechanism relevant for the specific iso-enzyme and metabolite structure(s). Such knowledge may not be readily available when assessing the metabolism of a new, unknown compound and generating this information would require a substantial effort. Thus, application of hepatocytes generally seems to offer

an advantage over the use of microsomes. However, the issue of product inhibition is only one of the pitfalls that may be encountered during *in vitro-in vivo* extrapolations of metabolism [21].

To date, scaling of *in vitro* data has relied entirely on the use of CLint and has assumed Michaelis-Menten kinetics. There are several chemicals whose metabolism cannot be explained with this model [67] and with others, diazepam for example, where different pathways require different models (appendix 7 in [66]. Failure to recognise this complication and adopt an alternative parameter (the utility of CLmax has been explored - [67] will lead to poor predictions. Another restriction to the commonly employed scaling strategy is the use of metabolite formation data. The use of substrate depletion-time profiles, and the inclusion of albumin in the incubation media might be considered. These methodological modifications can be made without concern to the validity of the parameters obtained for prediction purposes, as exemplified with diazepam and phenytoin [66].

Other kinetic considerations

Another possible cause for inappropriate assessment of metabolism by *in vitro* systems is related to the occurrence of unrealistic, high Kms in selected literature data examined for toluene [63] and parathion. This has been explained by the fact that the actual free substrate concentration in the *in vitro* system can be much lower than expected from the total amount of substrate that is present, due to the occurrence of binding of compounds to e.g. proteins. This problem occurs inconsistently and "normal" Km values for toluene are also reported. It seems not feasible to make conclusive remarks about this from the present results, due to the limited number of observations. In this respect, a possible follow-up of the present study would require a wider range of compounds to be considered.

Possible auto-induction of metabolism, i.e. increased metabolism rate of a compound induced by the compound itself, is presently not addressed. Auto-induction can become relevant in the case of (sub)chronic *in vivo* exposure, and will be reflected by an increased metabolism rate during exposure. This could be accounted for by exposing animals to the relevant compound for a selected time proceeding the isolation of hepatocytes or microsomes used for *in vitro* metabolism assessment of that compound. Although such studies have been reported *in vivo*, their design is usually limited to a single challenge dose making the results unsuitable for quantitative *in vitro-in vivo* extrapolations.

Possible sex- and age-specificity of metabolism is another issue that could not be addressed comprehensively within the present study, although its occurrence was infrequently observed, e.g. for caffeine [66]. Possible occurrence of sex- and age-specific metabolism is related to the iso-enzymes involved in the metabolism of the compounds [74]. A first approach could be made through an inventory of the knowledge on this aspect from the literature. The sex- and age-specificity of body composition is directly related to the previous issue. A high body fat content may decrease the availability of lipophilic compounds for a target tissue or for hepatic metabolism. We have attempted to account for age-specificity of localized body fat depots of rats by using an algorithm that describes body fat deposit size as a function of body weight. However, this information is presently available for only two rat strains; Sprague-Dawley and Fisher-344 [27].

In relation to the previously discussed role of fat deposit size, the issue of diffusion-limited fat-blood distribution is demonstrated in the case of parathion [66]. Although similar phenomena may also occur for lindane, phenytoin and diazepam, the lack of abundant data presently limits the discussion to parathion. Diffusion limitation causes an overestimation of fat concentrations at the early timepoints due to a delayed uptake in the fat compartment(s). As a result, concentrations in other tissues may be underestimated since the total mass balance of compound present in the body remains unchanged. Thus, estimates for actual target tissue concentrations at these timepoints may be too low. In addition, the resulting liver concentrations may be actually higher than estimated, resulting in an increased metabolism rate, provided that metabolism is not saturated. As we are currently not aware of non-animal techniques for quantification of fat-blood diffusion, the relevance of diffusion limitation may be tentatively investigated through sensitivity analysis of the model.

Assessment of extrahepatic metabolism is yet another issue that was presently not addressed. Although extrahepatic metabolism has been reported, e.g for diazepam in lung and kidney tissue [75], it has generally been found of minor significance. For compounds that express their toxicity through the parent compound, it may become relevant when the metabolic rate is in the same order of magnitude as the hepatic metabolism. For compounds that express their toxicity through bioactivation, even relatively small extrahepatic metabolism rates can become significant as it may lead to accumulation of toxic metabolites in the target tissue. It may possibly play a role for benzene in the bone marrow [76], and in the brain for toluene and parathion [77].

9.7.2 Dynamics

The second main goal of the present studies lies in the estimation of *in vivo* toxicity from *in vitro*-derived data, once the kinetics have been taken into account.

Prediction on the basis of in vitro vs in vivo data: replacement or reduction.

The results for lindane and acrylamide show that if a full *in vitro*-based kinetic model is not feasible, acute to (sub)chronic extrapolations through kinetic simulations may be used to assess the (sub)chronic toxicity of these compounds [66,68]. Although the outcome of the LOEL estimations relied, at least in part, on *in vivo* studies, a reduction in the use of animal models is achieved from the extrapolation of acute to (sub)chronic kinetics and application of the *in vitro* toxicity data.

Appropriate in vitro toxicity parameters.
The limitation of the toxicity estimates for caffeine, phenytoin and diazepam to acute exposure scenarios arises from the assumptions outlined in the introduction. Neuro-toxicity was assessed *in vitro* by determination of various endpoints after exposure through the culture medium for a fixed, continuous period of 72 hours. This gives the concentration-response information from which the concentration corresponding to a 20% effect is derived as a measure for the critical neurotic concentration (CNC). Since this CNC is used as a threshold for occurrence of the lowest observed effects, the estimated occurrence of effect depends directly on the actual presence of a compound in the target tissue. In cases where a compound accumulates in the target tissue over time, as for linden, the difference between acute and (sub)chronic Loess reflects the build-up of target tissue concentrations over time. If the half-life of a compound in the target tissue is smaller than the dosing frequency, this compound will not accumulate over time, and LOEL estimates will lead to identical values for acute and (sub)chronic exposure. In order to overcome this limitation, the half life of an effect must be known in addition to the half life of the compound that induces this effect. This requires knowledge of the *in vitro* effect as a function of both time and concentration, preferably including a post exposure observation period. Application of these considerations for acrylamide demonstrates the power of this approach [68]. Although it required extra research efforts, they seemed well justified by the results.

The presumptions that lead to the present study regarding the direct correlation between *in vitro* derived-CNCs and occurrence of LOELs *in vivo*, should also be considered from a stochastical point of view. By definition, the LOEL is the lowest exposure level causing a significant effect, either above or below control levels. Besides the theoretical arguments that can be raised against this presumption, statistical theory also implies that a LOEL (at a given level of significance, e.g. $p<0.05$) depends on the number of observations in the exposure group. In addition, the methods applied for effect assessment *in vivo* and *in vitro* may not have equal sensitivity to pick up effects due to differences in reproducibility. The benchmark dose approach is based on the 95% lower confidence limit of the estimated NOEL extrapolated from a dose- or concentration-response curve [78]. Several aspects of this approach could be incorporated into the presently attempted methods for *in vitro-in vivo* toxicity extrapolations, and are expected to lead to a better confidence in the outcome of future studies in this field.

Integration of in vitro test batteries and other non-animal studies.
The present results indicate that specific effects of the eight compounds were not always picked up by the *in vitro* neurotoxicity test battery. Besides the methodological limits for the volatile solvents benzene and toluene, the specific mechanisms for toxicity (or activity) of phenytoin, diazepam and, to a lesser extent parathion and caffeine, were not adequately reflected by the results of the test battery. From the issues discussed in section 3.2, we propose that additional test systems should be considered after a structural analysis of the compounds by a SAR-driven database such as DEREK [79]. A positive identification of structural alerts for specific toxicity such as AChE inhibition or interference with the GABA system, would offer a rationale for additional *in vitro* testing in systems that are explicitly designed for the relevant endpoints. Even then, it has to be realized that e.g. the GABA receptor may occur in multiple subtypes, and the inclusion of a single *in vitro* endpoint specifically relevant for (human) toxicity or activity will be difficult.

There are no straightforward rules for addressing the role of metabolic activation in the toxicity of compounds. Within the present study, the role of paraoxon in parathion toxicity was identified based on common knowledge from the literature. Some information was also available on the possible toxicity of metabolites of caffeine and diazepam [80,81]. However, assessment of the toxicity of these metabolites, including both kinetic and dynamic aspects, has to await a future study. In general, the comprehensive *in vitro* toxicity assessment for all metabolites of a compound may not be feasible. In order to anticipate on metabolic activation of unknown compounds, QSAR analysis can be applied to the outcome of *in vitro* biotransformation studies to direct the attention of the researcher to metabolites that may be relevant.

Interspecies extrapolation.
In the present study, estimation and evaluation of neurotoxicity were limited to the rat. Obviously, this is not the eventual species of interest for human risk assessment. We have limited ourselves to the rat due to the abundant availability of data for this species. Thus, the validity of the studied methodology could be evaluated as much as possible. From the lessons learned from these evaluations, kinetics should be the starting points for extrapolation from rats to humans. This may be motivated by the fact that data on human physiology are readily available from the literature. In addition, qualitative and quantitative differences in the metabolic pathways between the two spe-

cies may be accounted for by considering *in vitro* studies on biotransformation in human material. Results are most abundant on human microsomes, but hepatocyte studies have also been described. *In vivo* data on kinetic behaviour in humans are most abundant for pharmaceuticals like caffeine, phenytoin and diazepam. *In vivo* data on pesticides or industrial compounds like lindane and parathion will be more limited to situations where a reliable determination of the exposure of the individuals will likely be very difficult.

9.8 Conclusions from the ECITTS study

In summary, it may be concluded that the ECITTS study has generated encouraging results on the possible methodologies of risk assessment of chemicals on the basis of *in vitro* studies and computer simulations. Application of the *in vitro* neurotoxicity test battery, kinetic simulations and QSAR analysis have identified some key directions of future research. The need for time-concentration-response relationships, including post-exposure recovery, is one of the most pronounced findings. Statistical aspects of the CNC-LOEL/NOEL relationship may be improved through methods used in the Benchmark Dose approach. QSAR-driven activity analysis may identify additional *in vitro* assays for those types of toxicity that are no addressed through the endpoints of the test battery in its present form. QSAR-analysis is also to be considered for establishing algorithms for estimation of oral and dermal uptake of compounds. Further evaluation of *in vitro-in vivo* relationships for biotransformation requires extension of the number of com-pounds in future studies.

Finally, it has to be emphasized that the principal goals of the present study cover many fundamental aspects of toxicology and pharmacology. As such, the outcome of this study can only be considered as a basis for supporting further investigations in each of the respective fields that have previously been discussed.

9.9 A generic scheme for evaluating chemical toxicity

On the basis of the ECITTS results, a more generic scheme for the evaluation of a compound's local and/or systemic toxicity has been proposed by an ECVAM Task Force (82). This generic scheme can be described as an integrated decision-making strategy for toxicological evaluation, with the emphasis on the use of non-animal data, which takes into account earlier proposals for parallel and tiered approaches (a schematic representation of this scheme can be found in [82]). It incorporates existing knowledge (including physicochemical data), biokinetic considerations and toxicological test systems ranging from determination of basal cytotoxicity to highly specific target tissue assays. A prerequisite for the success of this scheme is the availability of appropriate, well-validated non-animal methods.

A key feature of the scheme is the presence of decision points, i.e. stages at which decisions are made with regard to further testing. In addition, the scheme allows for expert judgement to be made at different stages of the scheme for the purposes of hazard assessment (including classification and labelling). The proposed scheme consists of four stages:

1. assessments based on physicochemical properties and chemical functionality,
2. biokinetic modelling, including the modelling of biotransformation, tissue partition and transport, together with basal cytotoxicity testing,
3. the selection from a battery of specific cytotoxicity and cell-specific function toxicity tests in the case of high tissue concentrations, and
4. the selection from a battery of specific cytotoxicity tests, if indicated by historical data for related chemical structures, regulatory requirements, or by the intended usage of the chemical.

On the basis of the outcome of each stage, expert judgement would result in identification of toxic hazard and/or progression to the next stage of the scheme. Thus, the scheme can be used both for screening purposes and for generating more comprehensive toxicological profiles.

Stage I
In the first stage, chemical structure and any relevant physicochemical data (e.g. melting point) are taken into account. Some physicochemical parameters (e.g. log P) and chemical functionality (e.g. electrophilicity) can be determined from the chemical structure. These data are then used to predict toxicological properties by using appropriate QSAR models. Currently available models include those for the prediction of skin irritation and corrosivity [83,84,85], eye irritation [86], skin sensitisation [87] and mutagenicity [88], for specific classes of chemicals.

Stage II
Central to stage II is a biokinetic model, which describes the time course of the concentration of a chemical in various tissues of the body. Such models can be constructed for any animal species of interest, provided that the appropriate physiological parameters are available (e.g. blood flows, tissue size and composition). A comprehensive compilation of these parameters is provided by Brown et al [27]. Compound-specific parameters, such as tissue partition coefficients, can be calculated from physicochemical properties,

whereas parameters such as the rates of biotransformation and transport need to be determined with appropriate *in vitro* systems [89]. When bioactivation is identified as an important process, the biokinetics of any relevant metabolites also need to be incorporated. The integration of physicochemical properties and *in vitro* data into physiologically based biokinetic models is illustrated by DeJongh et al. [22], and by Houston & Carlile [21,90], respectively.

Also important at this stage is knowledge about the basal cytotoxicity of a chemical and any relevant metabolites, i.e. toxicity towards processes which are common to all cell types [91]. This can be determined using one of a number of basal cytotoxicity tests, such as the neutral red uptake (NRU) assay.

The output of biokinetic models is the prediction of concentration/time courses in different tissues, and the identification of tissues which concentrate the chemical. This information can be combined with the basal cytotoxicity data to make a prediction of the acute systemic toxicity of the chemical. Thus, chemicals which are potentially hazardous to specific tissues, can be identified. It may also be possible to predict non-specific effects, such as the accumulation of non-reactive lipophilic chemicals in biological membranes; this phenomenon is referred to as baseline toxicity, and manifests itself as a general "narcotic" effect in the nervous system [69].

Stage III

If the outcome of stage II indicates the presence of high concentrations of a chemical in a particular tissue, then the toxicity of the chemical in that tissue needs to be determined. Two forms of specific toxicity are recognised:

a) selective toxicity, in which some cell types are more sensitive than others; and
b) cell-specific function toxicity, in which the chemical affects events or structures which are unique to, or particularly dominant in, a specific cell type.

This could include effects which are critical to the organism as a whole, such as the inhibition of albumin production in hepatocytes, cytokine production or hormone production [91].

The outcome of the experiments carried out at this stage can be expressed as the ratio of the effective concentration for basal cytotoxicity to the effective concentration for the cell-specific toxicity. Ratios considerably greater than one would indicate specific target organ toxicity, and a requirement to determine a "no observed effect level" (NOEL). The choice of cell types is mainly determined on the basis of biokinetic considerations or information of a physicochemical nature for chemicals with similar characteristics.

Stage IV

Even when a chemical does not appear to accumulate in any specific tissue, or when its ratio of basal cytotoxicity to specific toxicity is not particularly high, there may still be other reasons for investigating more closely the tissue-specific effects of the chemical, e.g. to comply with particular regulatory requirements related to the expected usage of the chemical. In such cases, test systems could include tissue-specific tests similar to those used in Stage III, but they could also include tests for other toxicological endpoints, such as developmental toxicity and carcinogenicity. The outcome of this stage will be similar to the outcome of Stage III, i.e. the classification and prediction of systemic toxicity.

If a chemical cannot be evaluated toxicologically by applying these four stages, it may be necessary to conduct limited *in vivo* studies. However, the information gained in previous stages will enable such studies to be more focussed than they would have otherwise been, so they will indeed be limited. Thus, these *in vivo* studies can be regarded as true refinements in comparison with animal procedures based on current testing guidelines.

9.10 Concluding remarks

The toxicity of chemicals is determined by two main sets of characteristics: a) the mode of action and the resulting effects on the organism (dynamics); and b) the changes in concentration of the chemical with time, in various parts of the organism (biokinetics). Therefore, integrated testing strategies must combine the use of toxico-dynamic and biokinetic parameters.

First results of e.g. the ECITTS programme have shown the feasibility and some limitations of the possibilities to integrate non-animal data from different domains:

- physicochemical properties of a compound (and tits concomitant chemical functionalities);
- data on the kinetics (e.g. biotransformation data);
- data on the toxicodynamics (e.g. on the mechanisms of action, the effective concentrations in relevant *in vitro* systems).

A prerequisite for predicting a compound's toxicity with the necessary accuracy is the availability of such data, which in turn is relying on the availability of the relevant well-validated *in vitro* methods.

The use of an integrated, stepwise (decision-tree) procedure, even when it is not fully depending on non-animal data, has yet another advantage. It allows a more structured, transparant and efficient way of performing risk assessment. The further implementation of these schemes is an absolute necessity in the future development of toxicology and risk assessment sciences.

Acknowledgements

This project was financed by the Swedish National Board for Laboratory Animals (CFN), the European Commission via ECVAM (Contract No 11277-95-10-F1ED ISP NL), and by the Dutch Platform Alternatives to Animal Experiments (project 94-31).

9.11 References

1. Kroes R, Feron VJ. (1990). Toxicity testing: strategies and conduct. In: Clayson DB, Minro IC, Shubik P, Seenberg JA, (eds.) Progress in Predictive Toxicology. Amsterdam: Elsevier, pp 15-39.
2. OECD (1993). Guidance document for the development of OECD guidelines for the testing of chemicals. OECD Monograph No. 76. Paris: Organisation for Economic Cooperation and Development.
3. Anon. (1986). European Convention for the Protection of Vertebrate Animals used for Experi-men-tal and Other Scientific Purposes, 51 pp. Strassbourg: Council of Europe.
4. Russell WMS, Burch RL. (1959). The principles of humane experimental technique. London: Methuen & Co Ltd, London.
5. Anon. (1986). Council directive of 24 November 1986 on the approximation of laws, regula-tions and administrative provisions of the member states regarding the protection of animals used for experimental and other purposes (directive 86/609/EEC). Official Journal of the European Communities 29(L358): 1-29.
6. Frazier JM, Goldberg AM (1990). Alternatives to and reduction of animal use in biomedical research, education and testing. Altern. Lab. Anim. 18: 65-74.
7. Relius HW (1987). Extrapolation from animals to man: prediction, pitfalls and perspectives. Xenobiotica 17: 255-265.
8. Blaauboer BJ, Balls M, Barratt M, Casati S, Coecke S, Mohamed MK, Moore J, Rall D, Smith KR, Tennant R, Schwetz BA, Stokes WS, Younes M (1998). 13th Meeting of the Scientific Group on Methodologies for the Safety Evaluation of Chemicals (SGOMSEC): Alternative testing methodologies and conceptual issues. Environmental Health Perspectives 106: 413 415
9. Barratt MD (1995). The role of structure-activity relationships and expert systems in alternative strategies for the determination of skin sensitisation, skin corrosivity and eye irritation. Altern. Lab. Anim 23: 111-122.
10. Walum E, Balls M, Bianchi V, Blaauboer B, Bolcsfoldi G, Guillouzo A, Moore GA, Odland L, Reinhardt C, Spielmann H (1992). ECITTS: an integrated approach to the application of *in vitro* test systems to the hazard assessment of chemicals. Altern. Lab. Anim. 20: 406-428.
11. Blaauboer BJ, Balls M, Bianchi V, Bolcsfoldi G, Guil-louzo A, Moore GA, Odland L, Reinhardt CA, Spielmann H, Walum E (1994). The ECITTS integrated toxicity testing scheme: the application of *in vitro* test systems to the hazard assessment of chemicals. Toxicol. *in vitro* 8: 845-846.
12. Balls M, Bridges J, Southee J (eds.) (1991). Animals and Alternatives in Toxicology: Present Status and Future Prospects. Basingstoke: MacMillan Press.
13. Frazier JM, Goldberg AM (1990). Alternatives to and reduction of animal use in biomedical research, education and testing. Altern. Lab. Anim. 18: 65-74.

14. Flint OP (1990). *In vitro* toxicity testing: purpose, validation and strategy. Alt. Lab. Anim. 18: 11-18.
15. Frazier JM (ed) (1992). *In vitro* Toxicity Testing: Applications to Safety Evaluation. New York: Marcel Dekker Inc.
16. Blaauboer BJ, Wortelboer HM, Mennes WC (1990). The use of liver cell cultures derived from different mammalian species in *in vitro* toxicological studies: implementation in extrapolation models? Altern. Lab. Anim. 18: 251-258.
17. Yang RSH, Andersen ME(1994). Pharmacokinetics. In: Hodgson E, Levi PE (eds.). Introduction to Biochemical Toxicology. East Norwalk: Appleton and Lange. pp: 49-73.
18. Clewell HJ, Andersen ME (1986). A multiple dose-route physiological model for volatile chemicals using ACSL/PC. In: Cellier FD (ed.) Languages for Continuous simulation. San Diego: Society for computer simulation. p 95.
19. Blaauboer BJ, DeJongh J (1997) Application of *in vivo* data on toxicity and biokinetics for estimation of systemic toxicity: the ECITTS scheme In: van Zutphen LFM, Balls M (eds.). Animal Alternatives, Welfare and Ethics, proceedings of the 2nd world congress on alternatives and animal use in the life sciences, held in Utrecht, The Netherlands, 20-24 October 1996. Elsevier. Amsterdam, Lausanne, New York, Oxford, Shannon, Tokyo. pp. 707-721
20. Atterwill CK, Bruinink A, Drejer J, Duarte E, Abdulla EM, Meredith C, Nicotera P, Regan C, Rodrígez-Farré, Simpson MG, Smith R, Veronesi B, Vijverberg H, Walum E, Williams DC (1994). *In vitro* neurotoxicity testing. ECVAM Workshop Report 3. 22: 350-362.
21. Houston JB, Carlile DJ (1997). Prediction of hepatic clearnce from microsomes, hepatocytes, and liver slices. Drug Metab. Rev. 29: 891-922.
22. DeJongh J, Verhaar HJM and Hermens JLM (1997). A quantitative property-property relationship QPPR approach to estimate *in vitro* tissue-blood partition coefficients of organic chemicals in rats and humans. Arch. Toxicol. 72: 17-25.
23. Andersen ME (1991) Physiological modelling of organic compounds. Ann. Occup. Hyg. 35: 309-321.
24. Yang RS Andersen ME (1994). Pharmacokinetics. In: Introduction to biochemical toxicology (Hodgson E, Levi PE, eds.) p. 49. Appleton and Lange, Norwalk
25. Leung HW (1991). Development and utilization of physiologically based models for toxico-logical applications. J. Toxicol. Environ. Health 32: 247-267.
26. Clewell HJ, Andersen ME (1986). A multiple dose-route physiological model for volatile chemi--cals using ACSL/PC. In: Languages for Continuous simulation (Cellier FD, ed.). Society for computer simulation, San Diego, p. 95.
27. Brown R, Foran J, Olin S, Robinson D. Physiological parameter values for PBPK models. 1994, International Life Sciences Institute, and Risk Science Institute, Washington, USA.
28. Artursson P, Karlsson J (1991). Correlation between oral drug absorption in humans an apparent drug permeability coefficeints in human intestinal epithelial (CACO-2) cells. Biochem. Bio-phys. Res. Comm. 175: 880-885.
29. Friend DR (1992). *In vitro* skin permeation techniques. J. Contr. Release 18: 235-248.
30. Kao J, Patterson K, Hall J (1985). Skin penetration and metabolism of topically applied chemicalss in six mammalian species, including man: an *in vitro* studiy with benzo(a)pyrene and testosterone. Toxicol. Appl. Pharmacol. 81: 502-516.
31. De Lange J, van Eck P, Elliott GR, de Kort WL, Wolthuis OL (1992).The isolated blood perfused pig ear: an inexpensive and animal-saving model for skin penetration studies. J. Pharmacol. Toxicol. Meth. 27: 71-77.

32. Austel V, Kutter E (1983). Absorption, distribution and metabolism of drugs. In: Quantitative-structure activity relationships of drugs (Topliss JG, ed.), p.437, Academic Press, New York.
33. McDougal JN, Jepson GW, Clewell HJ, Gargas ML, Andersen ME (1990). Dermal absorption of organic chemical vapours in rats and humans. Fund. Appl. Toxicol. 14: 299-308.
34. Seydel JK, Schaper KJ (1982). Quantitative structure-pharmacokinetic relationships and drug design. Pharmac. Ther. 15: 131-182.
35. Sato A, Nakajima T (1979). A structure-activity relationship of some chlorinated hydrocarbons. Arch. Environ. Health; March/Apr., 69-75.
36. Perbellini L, Brugnone F, Caretta D, Maranelli G (1985). Partition Coefficients of some indus-trial aliphatic hydrocarbons (C5-C7) in blood and human tissues. Br. J. Ind. Med. 42: 162-167.
37. Fiserova-Bergerova V, Diaz ML (1986). Determination and prediction of tissue-gas partition coefficients. Int. Arch. Occup. Environ. Health 58: 75-87.
38. Gargas ML, Burgess RJ, Voisard DE, Cason GH, Andersen ME (1989). Partition coefficients of low-molecular-weight volatile chemicals in various liquids and tissues. Toxicol. Appl. Pharmacol. 98: 87-99.
39. Pacifici GM, Viani A (1992). Methods of determining plasma and tissue binding of drugs. Clin. Pharmacokinet. 23: 449-468.
40. Jepson GW, Hoover DK, Black RK, McCafferty JD, Mahle DA, Gearhart JM (1994). A parti-tion coefficient determination method for nonvolatile chemicals in biological tissues. Fund. Appl. Toxicol. 22: 519-524.
41. Bäärnhielm C, Dahlbäck H, Skanberg I (1986). *In vivo* pharmacokinetics of felodipine predicted from *in vitro* studies in rat, dog and man. Acta Pharmacol. Toxicol. 59: 113-122.
42. Gearhart JM, Jepson GW, Clewell H, Andersen ME, Conolly RB (1990). Physiologically based pharmacokinetic and pharmacodynamic model for the inhibition of acetylcholinesterase by diisopropylfluorophosphate. Toxicol. Appl. Pharmacol. 106: 295-310.
43. Toftgard R, Haaparanta T, Eng L, Halpert J (1986). Rat lung and liver microsomal cytochrome P-450 isoenzymes involved in the hydroxylation of n-hexane. Biochem. Pharmacol. 35: 3733-3738.
44. Hildebrand RL, Andersen ME, Jenkins LJ (1981). Prediction of *in vivo* kinetic constants from kinetic constants measured *in vitro*. Fund. Appl. Toxicol. 1: 403-409.
45. Kedderis GL, Carfagna MA, Held SD, Batra R, Murphy JE, Gargas ML (1993). Kinctic analysis of furan biotransformation by F-344 rats *in vivo* and *in vitro*. Toxicol Appl. Pharmacol. 123: 274-282.
46. Carlile DJ, Zomorodi K, Houston JB (1997) Scaling factors to relate drug metabolic clearance in hepatic microsomes, isolated hepatocytes, and the intact liver: studies with induced livers involving diazepam. Drug. Metab. Dispos. 25: 903-11
47. Gargas ML, Seyboldt PG, Andersen ME (1988). Modeling the tissue solubilities and metabolic rate constant (Vmax) of halogenated methanes, ethanes and ethylenes. Toxicol. Lett. 43: 235-256.
48. Atterwill C, Johnston H, Thomas SM (1992). Models for the *in vitro* assessment of neurotoxicity in the nervous system in relation to xenobiotic and neurotrophic factor-mediated events. Neurotoxicology 13: 39-54.
49. Walum E (1992). Studies of neurotoxicity in cellular models. In: *In vitro* alternatives to animal pharmaco-toxicology. Farmaindustria, Serie Científica, Madrid, . pp. 205-237.
50. Veronesi B (1992). *In vitro* screening batteries for neurotoxicants. Neurotoxicology 13: 185-196

51. Ekwall B. and 32 co-authors (1998). MEIC Evaluation of Acute Systemic Toxicity. Part VI. Prediction of human toxicity by rodent LD50 values and results from 61 *in vitro* tests 26: 617-658.
52. Nordin-Andersson M, Forsby A, Heldring N, DeJongh J, Kjellstrand P, Walum E (1998). Neurite degeneration in differentiated human neuroblastoma cells. Toxicol. *in vitro* 5: 557-560
53. Forsby A, Pilli F, Bianchi V,Walum E (1995). Determination of critical cellular neurotoxic con-centrations in human neuroblastoma (SH-SY5Y) cell cultures. Altern. Lab. Anim.11: 800-811.
54. Dunlop XX (1983). Protein turnover in brain: syntheis and degradation. In: Handbook of Neuro-chemistry, Ch. 5. Metabolic turnover in the nervous system. Plenum Press, New York. pp. 25-63
55. Andres M, Forsby A, Walum E (1997). Polygodial-induced noradrenaline release in human neuroblastoma SH-SY5Y cells. Toxicol. *In vitro* 11: 509-511.
56. Verity MA. (1992). Ca2+-dependent processes as mediators of neurotoxicity. Neurotoxicology 13: 139-148.
57. McConkey DJ, Orrenius S (1998). The role of calcium in the regulation of apoptosis. J. Leukocyte Biol. 59: 775-783.
58. Pörn-Ares IM, Ares MPS, Orrenius S (1998). Calcium signalling and the regulation of apoptosis. Toxicol. *In vitro* 12: 539-543.
59. Murphy NP, Vaughhan PFT, Ball SG, McCormack JG (1991). The cholinergic regulation of intracellular calcium in the human neuroblastoma, SH-SY5Y. J. Neurochem. 57: 2116-2123.
60. Toselli M, Masetto S, Rossi P, Taglietti V (1991). Characterization of a voltage-dependent calcium current in the human neuroblastoma cell line SH-SY5Y during differentiation. Eur. J. Neurosci. 3: 514-522.
61. Påhlman S, Ruusala AI, Abrahamsson L, Mattsson MEK, Esscher T (1984). Retinoic acid-induced differentiation of cultured human neuroblastoma cells: a comparison with phorbol-ester-induced differentiation. Cell Diff. 14: 135-144.
62. DeJongh J and Blaauboer BJ (1996). *In vitro*-based and *in vivo* based simulations of benzene uptake and metabolism in rats. Altern. Lab. Anim. 24: 179-190.
63. DeJongh J and Blaauboer BJ (1996). Simulation of toluene kinetics in the rat by a physiologically based pharmacokinetic model with application of biotranformation parameters derived independently *in vitro* and *in vivo*. Fund. Appl. Toxicol. 32: 260-268.
64. DeJongh J and Blaauboer BJ (1997). Simulation of lindane kinetics in rats. Toxico-logy 122: 1-9.
65. Murrey M and Butler AM (1994). Hepatic biotransformation of parathion : role of cytochrome P450 in NADPH- and NADH-mediated microsomal oxidation *in vitro*. Chem. Res. Toxicol. 9: 611-619.
66. Blaauboer BJ, DeJongh J, Forsby A, Heldring N, Nordin Andersson M, Guillouzo A, Houston JB, Witherow L, Odland L, Beckman M, Walum E, Combes R, Clothier R (1998). An integrated approach to the prediction of systemic toxicity using computer-based biokinetic models and biological *in vitro* test methods: A prevalidation study based on the ECITTS project. Report for ECVAM, Environment Institute of the EU Joint Research Centre, Ispra, Italy. 38 pp and 24 appendices.
67. Witherow LE, Houston JB (1999). Sigmoidal kinetics of CYP3A substrates: an approach for scaling dextromethorphan metabolism in hepatic microsomes and isolated hepatocytes to predict *in vivo* clearance in rat. J. Pharmacol. Exp. Ther. 290: 58-65

68. DeJongh J, Nordin-Andersen M, Ploeger BA, Forsby A (1999). Estimation of systemic toxicity of acrylamide by integration of *in vitro* data with kinetic simulations. Toxicol. Appl. Pharmacol. 158: 261-268.
69. DeJongh J, Verhaar HJ, Hermens JL (1998) Role of kinetics in acute lethality of nonreactive volatile organic compounds (VOCs). Toxicol-Sci. 45: 26-32
70. Ramsey JC, Andersen ME (1984). A physiologically based description of the inhalation pharma--co-kinetics of styrene in rats and humans. Toxicol. Appl. Pharmacol. 73: 159-175.
71. EPA (1992). Dermal exposure assessment: Principles and applications. EPA interim report EPA/600/8-91/011B, EPA , Washington DC.
72. Poulin P, Krishnan K (1996). A mechanistic algorithm for predicting blood:air partition coefficients of organic chemicals with the consideration of reversible binding in hemoglobin. Toxicol. Appl. Pharmacol. 136: 131-137.
73. Woodruff TJ, Bois FY, Auslander D, Spear RC (1992). Structure and parameterization of pharmacokinetic models: their impact on model predictions. Risk Anal. 12: 189-201.
74. Imaoka S, Fujita S, Funae Y (1991). Age-dependent expression of cytochrome P450s in rat liver. Bioch. Biophys. Acta 1097: 187-192.
75. Igari Y, Sugiyama Y, Sawada Y, Iga T, Hanano M (1983). Prediction of diazepam disposition in the rat and man by a physiologically based pharmacokinetic model. J. Pharmacokin. Biopharm. 11: 577-593.
76. Travis CC, Quillen JL, Arms AD (1990). Pharmacokinetics of benzene. Toxicol. Appl. Pharmacol. 99: 400-420.
77. Chambers JE, Chambers HW, Snawder JE (1991). Target site bioactivation of the neurotoxic organo-phosphorus insecticide parathion in partially hepatectomized rats. Life Sci. 48: 1023-1029.
78. Crump KS (1995). Calculation of benchmark doses from continuous data. Risk Anal. 15: 79-89.
79. Judson PN (1992). QSAR and expert systems in prediction of biological activity. Pestic. Sci. 36: 155-160.
80. Wilkinson JM, Pollard I (1993). Accumulation of theophylline, theobromine and paraxanthine in the fetal rat brain following a single oral dose of caffeine. Dev. Brain Res. 75: 193-199.
81. Seddon T, Michelle I, Chenery, R.J (1989). Comparitive drug metabolism of diazepam in hepatocytes isolated from man, rat, monkey and dog. Biochem. Pharmacol. 38: 1657-65.
82. Blaauboer BJ, Barratt MD, Houston JB (1999). The integrated use of alternative methods in toxicological risk evaluation. ECVAM Integrated Testing Strategies Task Force Report 1. Alternatives to Laboratory Animals 27: 229-237.
83. Barratt, M.D. (1996). Quantitative structure-activity relationships (QSARs) for skin corrosivity of organic acids, bases and phenols: principal components and neural network analysis of extended datasets. Toxicol. *in vitro* 10: 85-94.
84. Barratt, M.D. (1996). Quantitative structure-activity relationships for skin irritation and corrosivity of neutral and electrophilic organic chemicals. Toxicol. *in vitro* 10: 247-256.
85. Barratt, M.D. (1997). QSARS for the eye irritation potential of neutral organic chemicals. Toxicol. *in vitro* 11: 1-8.
86. Barratt, M.D., Dixit, M.B. & Jones, P.A. (1996). The use of *in vitro* cytotoxicity measurements for the prediction of the skin corrosivity potential of acids: a QSAR method. Toxicol. *in vitro* 10: 283-290.
87. Cronin, M.T. & Basketter, D.A. (1994). Multivariate analysis of a skin sensitization database. SAR and QSAR in Environmental Research 2: 159-179.

88. Benigni, R., Andreoli, C. & Giuliani, A. (1994). QSAR models for both mutagenic potency and activity: application to nitroarenes and aromatic amines. Environm. Mol. Mutagenesis 24: 208-219.
89. Arturrson, P. & Borchardt, R. (1997). Intestinal drug absorption and metabolism in cell cultures: caco-2 and beyond. Pharmac. Res. 14: 1655-1660.
90. Houston, J.B. & Carlile, D.J. (1997a). Incorporation of *in vitro* drug metabolism data into physiologically-based pharmacokinetic models. Toxicol. *in vitro* 11: 473-478.
91. Seibert, H., Balls, M., Fentem, J.H., Bianchi, V., Clothier, R.H., Dierickx, P.J., Ekwall, B., Garle, M.J., Gómez-Lechón, M.J., Gribaldo, L., Gülden, M., Liebsch, M., Rasmussen, E., Roguet, R., Shivrastava, R. & Walum, E. (1996). Acute toxicity testing *in vitro* and the classification and labelling of chemicals. The report and recommendations of ECVAM workshop 16. Altern. Lab. Anim. 24: 499-510.